CONCISE GUIDE TO

# Somatic Therapies in Psychiatry

American Psychiatric Press

# CONCISE GUIDES

Robert E. Hales, M.D.
*Series Editor*

Eve Nelson Shapiro
*Project Editor*

CONCISE GUIDE TO

# Somatic Therapies in Psychiatry

Laurence B. Guttmacher, M.D.

Director, Somatic Therapies Service
Director, Residency Training
Department of Psychiatry
University of Rochester
School of Medicine and Dentistry
Rochester, New York

American Psychiatric Press, Inc.

1400 K Street, N.W.
Washington, DC 20005

Manufactured in the United States of America

First Edition 88 89 90 91 6 5 4 3 2 1

The paper used in this publication meets the minimum requirements of American National Standard for Information Sciences—Permanence of Paper for Printed Library Materials, ANSI Z39.48-1984. ∞™

**Library of Congress Cataloging-in-Publication Data**

Guttmacher, Laurence B., 1947-
Concise guide to somatic therapies in psychiatry / Laurence B. Guttmacher. — 1st ed.
p. cm. — (Concise guides / American Psychiatric Press)
Includes bibliographies and index.
ISBM 0-88048-122-6 (alk. paper)
1. Psychopharmacology. I. Title. II. Series: Concise guides (American Psychiatric Press)
[DNLM: 1. Mental Disorders—drug therapy. 2. Psychotropic Drugs—therapeutic use. WM 402 G985c]
RC483.G88 1988
615′.78—dc19
DNLM/DLC
for Library of Congress 88-3285
CIP

This book is for Terry and Joshua, who showed remarkable tolerance and love during the very strange hours that this work demanded.

**Note:** The author has worked to ensure that all information in this book concerning drug dosages, schedules, and routes of administration is accurate as of the time of publication and consistent with standards set by the U.S. Food and Drug Administration and the general medical community. As medical research and practice advance, however, therapeutic standards may change. For this reason and because human and mechanical errors sometimes occur, we recommend that readers follow the advice of a physician who is directly involved in their care or the care of a member of their family.

The opinions or assertions contained herein are the private ones of Dr. Hales and are not to be construed as official or reflecting the views of the Department of Defense, the Uniformed Services University of the Health Sciences, Walter Reed Army Medical Center, or the Department of the Army. This book was prepared in the author's private capacity. Neither government-financed time nor supplies were used in connection with this project.

# CONTENTS

# Acknowledgments

Real appreciation goes to Rosemarie Oppelt for her assistance with manuscript preparation and to Leon Eisenberg, M.D., and Thomas Williams, M.D., Ph.D., whose critical reading of early drafts made a great deal of difference.

# INTRODUCTION

**to the *American Psychiatric Press Concise Guides***

The *American Psychiatric Press Concise Guides* series provides, in a most accessible format, practical information for psychiatrists—and especially for psychiatry residents and medical students—working in such varied treatment settings as inpatient psychiatry services, outpatient clinics, consultation/liaison services, and private practice. The *Concise Guides* are meant to complement the more detailed information to be found in lengthier psychiatry texts.

The *Concise Guides* address topics of greatest concern to psychiatrists in clinical practice. The books in this series contain a detailed Table of Contents, along with an index, tables, and charts, for easy access; and their size, designed to fit into a lab coat pocket, makes them a convenient source of information. The number of references has been limited to those most relevant to the material presented.

The selection and proper use of psychopharmacologic agents and electroconvulsive therapy is an important clinical concern that every practitioner must face. Laurence B. Guttmacher, M.D., has a wealth of academic and clinical experience in educating residents about their use. He begins this *Concise Guide to Somatic Therapies in Psychiatry* by presenting an approach to pharmacologic decision-making, and by highlighting 19 rules that psychiatrists should consider in their general approach to medication usage. Dr. Guttmacher also summarizes some basic pharmacological principles pertinent to psychoactive medications. This *Concise Guide* emphasizes those somatic treatments used to treat the most common disorders: antipsychotics, antidepressants, lithium, carbamazepine, electroconvulsive therapy, and anxiolytics.

Of particular interest to psychiatrists are the effects of aging upon a medication's pharmacokinetics. Dr. Guttmacher includes a chapter on geriatric psychopharmacology that summarizes the use of psychotropic medications in this population, and informs physicians about the management of agitation and dementia. He also includes a chapter on the psychopharmacologic treatment of other psychiatric disorders of special clinical significance: aggression, alcoholism, cocaine abuse, eating disorders, panic disorders, and others.

This book is organized to provide the physician with basic and applied information needed to make treatment decisions. The *Concise Guide to Somatic Therapies in Psychiatry* is an accessible, easy to use reference that can be readily available when making pharmacological recommendations. Dr. Guttmacher has written an outstanding, compact, and portable guide.

Robert E. Hales, M.D.
Series Editor
*American Psychiatric Press Concise Guides*

# INTRODUCTION



This text provides an overview of psychopharmacology. It is intended for those who are beginning to work in the area and for others who might be seeking a quick refresher.

These pages contain many facts. However, if this book succeeds, it will convey something more important: It will teach the reader how to think like a psychopharmacologist. This skill is transferable to other branches of medicine and nonpharmacologic therapeutics as well. The logic and the approach should be the same whether one is choosing an antipsychotic, determining which antibiotic to use for pneumonia, or even deciding whether to institute family or individual psychotherapy.

## ■ APPROACHES TO PHARMACOLOGICAL DECISION MAKING

***Document those signs and symptoms that are amenable to pharmacotherapy and are useful indicators of the patient's overall clinical state.***

Clinicians should document in writing the signs and symptoms they are targeting before instituting treatment. Failure to do this is a common clinical error. If this is not done, the physician may be confronted several weeks later with a completely new set of problems and will not be sure if the difficulties are iatrogenic or are part of the original illness. Start by picking several target behaviors and assess the severity of the problems before writing the first prescription. The simple approach is, for example, to target early morning awakening, anorexia, diurnal variation, and suicide ideation and rate them at 70, 80, 65, and 55 respectively, with 100 representing the maximal possible intensity. Alternatively, standard rating scales such as the Hamilton Depression Scale or the Brief Psychiatric Rating Scale could be used serially to monitor progress (1, 2).

***Establish a meaningful set of differential diagnoses.***

A patient can present to the emergency room with exactly the same findings from ingesting cocaine, experiencing schizophrenia, or having meningitis. Haloperidol might help the resultant behavior with all three, but it would probably be unnecessary for the patient who ingested cocaine since the psychosis is likely to resolve on its own. In the case of meningitis, haloperidol would certainly be a less desirable treatment than penicillin. Primary psychiatric differentials are greatly facilitated through the use of structured diagnostic interviews like the Structured Clinical Interview for *DSM-III-R* (3). At a minimum, the *Diagnostic and Statistical Manual of Mental Disorders, Third Edition, Revised (DSM-III-R)* (4) should be routinely consulted.

***Obtain a detailed drug history.***

If a patient has responded to imipramine during two previous episodes, there is no reason to begin nortriptyline. If a patient previously has been dystonic when challenged with haloperidol, the clinician should use another antipsychotic or should prophylactically administer an anticholinergic. It is important to obtain family histories of response or toxicity to particular agents, especially if there is no better way to decide among various agents.

***Do not begin drug treatment before completing steps one through three. The only exception should be for frank emergencies, and these are decidedly rare.***

There is almost always time to stop and think. This requires the ability to resist internal pressure, as well as pressure from nursing staff, to jump in and do "something." Remember that "doing something" without a well-thought-out rationale may lead to complications and serious consequences.

***If a patient is taking clinically significant doses of medication that are not causing toxicity when first encountered, then continue the medication while you are performing your initial evaluation.***

Failure to attend to this principle leads to confusion between withdrawal effects and undertreated primary illness.

***Whenever possible, avoid changing more than one variable at a time.***

This rule is generally honored in the breach, since it is rarely possible to isolate variables this cleanly; we frequently take patients away from work, admit them, begin family and activities therapy, and start an antipsychotic simultaneously. Much of this cannot and should not be avoided, but it is almost always possible

TABLE 1. **Average Wholesale Price for Pharmacists**

| Drug | Dose | Cost to Pharmacist |
|---|---|---|
| **Antipsychotics** | | |
| Chlorpromazine | 100mg | $ .04 |
| Fluphenazine decanoate | 1 ml/syringe[a] | 7.76 |
| Fluphenazine HCl | 2.5 mg | .37 |
| Haloperidol | 2 mg | .27 |
| Loxapine | 10 mg | .33 |
| | 25 mg | .50 |
| Mesoridazine | 25 mg | .28 |
| Molindone | 10 mg | .26 |
| Thioridazine | 100 mg | .12 |
| Thiothixene | 5 mg | .27 |
| Trifluoperazine | 5 mg | .09 |
| **Anticholinergics** | | |
| Benztropine | 2 mg | .04 |
| Diphenhydramine | 25 mg | .01 |
| **Antidepressants** | | |
| Amitriptyline | 150 mg | .07 |
| Amoxapine | 100 mg | .65 |
| Desipramine | 150 mg | 1.18 |
| Doxepin | 150 mg | .33 |
| Fluoxitene | 40 mg | 2.20 |
| Imipramine | 150 mg | .09 |
| Maprotiline | 150 mg | .88 |
| Nortriptyline | 75 mg | .71 |
| Phenelzine | 60 mg | .49 |
| Tranylcypromine | 30 mg | .57 |
| Trazodone | 300 mg | 1.45 |
| **Benzodiazepines and related compounds** | | |
| Alprazolam | 1 mg | .36 |
| Buspirone | 5 mg | .49 |
| Clonazepam | 1 mg | .22 |
| Diazepam | 5 mg | .05 |
| Flurazepam | 30 mg | .16 |
| Lorazepam | 1 mg | .09 |
| Temazepam | 30 mg | .25 |
| Triazolam | .5 mg | .26 |
| **Lithium carbonate** | 300 mg | .03 |
| Lithobid | 300 mg | .08 |

From American Druggist Blue Book, 1986-7 Edition, New York, Hearst.
[a] 25 mg, normally a two-week supply.

actively in treatment. The ideal physician is willing to devote considerable energy and time toward forging a relationship with the patient and his or her family, is able to hear feedback from them, is willing to educate them about the medicine, and is able to see medication as part of a larger treatment program.

***Consider cost when prescribing.***

One antidepressant may cost eight or nine times another. There may be special indications for an expensive drug's use, but there are few reasons to routinely use such a compound as a first-line agent. The patents for many psychotropics are just now expiring, so generic alternatives are becoming available. Each chapter will include a table listing which drugs are available generically. There are few convincing data to suggest significant differences in bioequivalence among various preparations in psychiatry, with the exception of medications for children. If a stable patient deteriorates, every effort should be made to learn whether a new generic drug was used, but such instances are rare.

Table 1 lists the cost to the pharmacist for some psychotropics. The cost to the patient will be higher once the pharmacy adds its markup. Prices will vary significantly for a drug when its patent protection ends and competition develops from generic preparations.

***Avoid polypharmacy.***

There is never any reason to give more than one drug from a particular class. There are, however, times when more than one class of drugs needs to be prescribed. Toxicity is often additive within a drug class, but desirable effects are not. For instance, all antipsychotics act by blocking the dopamine receptor, but they differ from one another in respect to which other receptors they affect. These other receptors cause much of the toxicity. Adding a second antipsychotic will only lead to unnecessary toxicity, which could be avoided simply by increasing one drug to a more appropriate level of dopamine blockade. This will become clearer when we discuss mechanisms of action in each chapter.

***Never use a fixed-combination drug.***

Fixed-combination drugs are allegedly constructed to enhance patient compliance. In fact, they may do the opposite. Generally, the constituents are present in such small doses that many pills would have to be taken to achieve the desired effect. Moreover, the prices of fixed-combination drugs are high. Most important, there is great loss in terms of flexibility; one cannot raise and lower the combined medications independently. A psychotic depression may require an antipsychotic and an antidepressant initially, but the antipsychotic should be lowered as the psychosis clears whereas the antidepressant should be maintained. Such a manipulation would be impossible with a fixed-combination drug.

***Dealing with an acute episode is different from prophylaxis.***

Electroconvulsive therapy (ECT) is the most effective treatment for an acute episode of depression, yet it has little demonstrated efficacy for the prevention of relapse. Lithium is effective for the prevention of recurrent unipolar depression but has relatively little to offer as an acute antidepressant.

***Don't try to learn about all the psychotropics.***

There are simply too many of them. Pick a smaller group and become comfortable with them. Thorough knowledge of four antipsychotics, three antidepressants, two benzodiazepines, one anticholinergic, and lithium should suffice for almost all patients.

***Maintain a healthy skepticism of new products and prescription trends.***

Jeste coined the "Law of the New Drug" when he pooled the studies of deanol, a cholinergic agonist, in the treatment of tardive dyskinesia (6). In the first year, 100% of studies reported positive results; after that, there was a steady decline until the fifth year, when all studies reported negative results. You should expect to be assaulted by advertising for every new drug, but beware of this. Remember that the two new psychotropics of 1986, nomifensine and bupropion, were withdrawn within months of marketing because of seizures and hemolytic anemia.

***There are no rules.***

All rules are based on populations of patients. Individual patients may well be outliers. The population of manic patients probably require lithium levels of 0.8–1.5 acutely, but individual patients may be best treated with levels of 0.3 or 2.0.

## ■ LEGAL ISSUES

Many of the treatments suggested in this book go beyond indications approved by the Food and Drug Administration (FDA). Use of imipramine in panic disorder or carbamazapine with bipolar patients are well-accepted therapies within the psychiatric community, but these indications are not specifically approved by the FDA. It is perfectly appropriate and defensible to use such treatments since they are well within community standards. It is important, however, to document your rationale for doing so. The most effective actions to prevent litigation are forming a good relationship with your patient, obtaining meaningful informed consent, documenting carefully what you have done, and behaving responsibly.

Unless otherwise noted, doses suggested are for average-sized, medically intact adults. No mention will be made of children or adolescents, and geriatric patients will be addressed in a separate section.

## ■ BASIC PHARMACOLOGY

### *KINETICS*

*The effective amount of a drug* reflects a dynamic equilibrium among absorption, distribution, metabolism, excretion, and, for psychiatry, the ability to cross the blood–brain barrier. Understanding these concepts will allow individualization of drug regimens to reflect changes with the aging process, drug interactions, or many physical impairments.

*Gastric absorption* is increased on an empty stomach, since direct mucosal contact is possible. Most psychoactive drugs are weak bases and are therefore best absorbed at the higher pH of the jejunum. Empty stomachs accelerate gastric emptying, which leads to more rapid contact with the area where most absorption occurs. The net result is that empty stomachs are associated with rapid onset of action. Rapid onset is not always desirable. Some drugs are embedded in a relatively nonabsorbable material in an attempt to slow absorption and provide a more gradual, smoother onset. Most drugs diffuse into the body. This process is facilitated by small, nonionized, lipid soluble molecules. Note that these are the same factors that are predictive of lipophilicity and of crossing the blood–brain barrier. It therefore follows that most psychoactive compounds are rapidly absorbed.

*The volume of distribution* is a theoretical construct defined as the amount of the drug in the body divided by the amount of the drug in plasma. Very lipophilic drugs, which is to say most psychoactive compounds, have large volumes of distribution. This is associated with a long half-life.

*The distribution phase* is the dispersion of the drug into tissue. Only free, unbound drugs will cross cell membranes. Psychotropics are highly bound to plasma proteins, notably albumin and glycoprotein. Only a small percentage of the drug is therefore available to the site of action, the brain.

*The blood–brain barrier* is not a specifiable place, but rather a functional system. Many drugs can be at high concentration peripherally and low level in the brain, or vice versa. This distinction is accounted for by the blood–brain barrier. Even though blood flow in the brain is remarkably high, drugs are slow to penetrate because brain capillaries lack the fenestrations seen peripherally and brain parenchyma is tightly packed, with little extracellular fluid.

*With the notable exception of lithium, most psychotropics are metabolized hepatically.* In some instances, the drug's effects are dependent on this since only the metabolites are psychoactive. In other cases, metabolism may be a part of clearing the drug from the body. Metabolism may also be complicated by a number of factors. The first-pass effect can be of major importance; 90% of fluphenazine HCl is metabolized before reaching the systemic circulation. This is why so many intramuscular (IM) preparations are more potent on a mg-per-mg basis than their oral congeners. Some drugs may stimulate hepatic enzymes responsible for their own degradation or that of other drugs. Patients on benzodiazepines will require more barbiturate prior tc ECT. Carbamazepine induces hepatic enzymes in a predictable fashion, so that levels dip after three to five weeks on the drug.

A drug's clearance reflects how it is removed from the body—this is one of the determinants of a drug's half-life. There are multiple half-lives, and imprecise speech often obscures which is being described. The *plasma half-life* is a measure of how long it takes to remove half of a drug from plasma, is the easiest to measure, and is therefore most commonly used. The *biological half-life* is that time necessary to remove half of a drug from the body. The *pharmacological half-life* is the time necessary to halve a drug's pharmacological effect. It is important to realize that drugs with long half-lives will take a long time to reach steady state and a long time to be cleared. Steady state is reached in about four to five half-lives. Dosage intervals less than two-thirds the half-life will be associated with minimal fluctuation in level once steady state is reached.

## THE NEURON AND SITES OF ACTION

Figure 1 represents a pair of idealized neurons. A neurotransmitter is synthesized in the presynaptic neuron, transported down the axon, and stored in presynaptic vesicles, which can be extravasated, dumping the transmitter into the synaptic cleft. Here the transmitter can latch onto receptors, which can be either presynaptic or postsynaptic. The presynaptic receptors are typically autoreceptors that regulate further synthesis and the release of more transmitter. The postsynaptic receptor will effect some response, frequently through the use of a second messenger. The effects of the transmitter will end in one of three ways: enzymatic degradation, diffusion, or reuptake into the presynaptic cell.

There are two determinants of receptor occupancy: a) the affinity of the receptor for the ligand and b) the amount of the

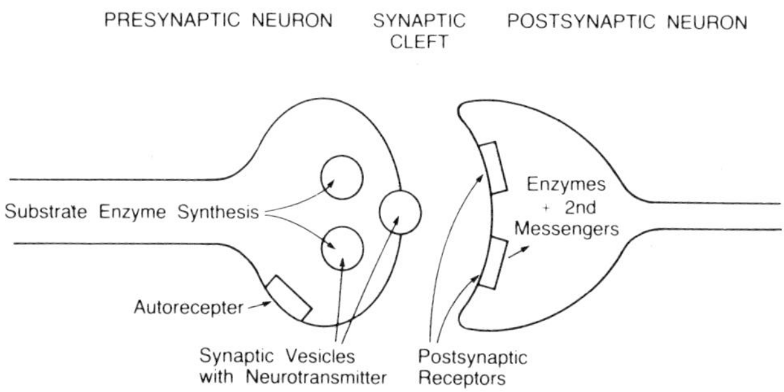


FIGURE 1. **The Neuron and Sites of Action.**

ligand in relation to the number of receptors. Receptors are in a state of dynamic equilibrium. The rate of synthesis for most is fixed, but the rate of degradation varies widely. Typical half-lives are in the range of 10 to 100 hours.

Ligands may be agonists or antagonists. Agonists effect a biological response. Partial agonists have weak biologic activity and compete for binding, but produce less of a response than a full agonist. Noncompetitive antagonists fully occupy receptors but produce no response. Binding is irreversible and no agonist will bind, no matter how high the concentration. The effect is to shift the drug response curve to the right, depressing the maximum possible response. Competitive antagonists, by contrast, can be overcome by sufficiently high concentrations of an agonist. Here the curve is shifted to the right (see Figure 2). The $ED_{50}$ is that dose of a drug that will effect half the maximal drug response.

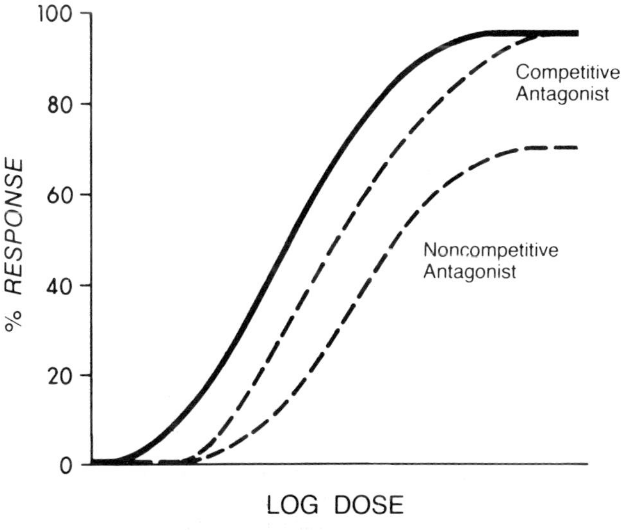


FIGURE 2. **Drug Response Curves for Competitive and Noncompetitive Antagonists.**

Denervation hypersensitivity occurs after prolonged occupation of a receptor by an antagonist. More receptors are created and there is an increase in the avidity of the receptor for the ligand. This increase in receptor number and affinity is referred to as *up-regulation*. The opposite situation—a decrease in the number of receptors and in affinity for the ligand—is referred to as *down-regulation*.

## ■ REFERENCES


1. Hamilton M: Development of a rating scale for primary depressive illness. Br J Soc Clin Psychol 1967; 6:278-296
2. Overall JE, Gorham DR: The Brief Psychiatric Rating Scale. Psychol Rep 1962; 10:799-812
3. Spitzer RL, Williams JBW, Gibbon M: Structured Clinical Interview for DSM-III-R. New York State Psychiatric Institute, Biometrics Research Department, 722 W. 168th St., NY, NY 10032
4. American Psychiatric Association: Diagnostic and Statistical Manual of Mental Disorders, Third Edition, Revised. Washington, DC, American Psychiatric Association, 1987
5. Blackwell B: The drug defaulter. Clin Pharmacol Ther 1972; 13:841-848
6. Jeste D, Wyatt RJ: Therapeutic strategies against tardive dyskinesia. Arch Gen Psychiatry 1982; 39:803-816


## ■ ANNOTATED GENERAL REFERENCES


1. Bassuk EL, Schoonover SC, Gelenberg AJ: The Practitioner's Guide to Psychoactive Drugs. New York, Plenum, 1984. A good basic, spiral-bound psychopharmacology reference.
2. Bochner F, Carruthers G, Kampmann J, et al: Handbook of Clinical Pharmacology. Boston, Little, Brown, 1983. A handy paperback edition on basic pharmacology.
3. Cooper JR, Bloom FE, Roth RH: The Biochemical Basis of Neuropharmacology. New York, Oxford University Press, 1987. An amazingly well written review of basic transmitter and receptor work.
4. Fink M: Convulsive Therapy: Theory and Practice. New York, Raven Press, 1979. *The* reference on ECT.
5. Guy W: ECDEU Assessment Manual for Psychopharmacology. Washington, DC, U.S. Department of Health, Education and Welfare, 1976. A wonderful compendium of rating scales.
6. Hales RE, Frances AJ (eds): Psychiatry Update: The American Psychiatric Association Annual Review (Volume 6). Washington,

DC, American Psychiatric Press, 1987. See section six for an excellent treatment of toxicities and interactions.

7. Jefferson JW, Greist JH, Ackerman DL, et al: Lithium Encyclopedia for Clinical Practice (second edition). Washington, DC, American Psychiatric Press, 1987. A masterful compendium of all matters relating to lithium.
8. Klein DF, Gittelman R, Quitkin F, et al: Diagnosis and Drug Treatment of Psychiatric Disorders: Adults and Children. Baltimore, Williams & Wilkins, 1980. An excellent basic text that could stand updating.
9. Meltzer HY (ed): Psychopharmacology: The Third Generation of Progress. New York, Raven Press, 1987. Multiple authored and therefore erratic, but still an excellent library reference.
10. Rizack MA, Hillman CDM: The Medical Letter Handbook of Adverse Drug Interactions. New Rochelle, NY, The Medical Letter, 1985. A wonderful place to look for troublesome interactions.
11. Salzman C: Clinical Geriatric Psychopharmacology, New York, McGraw-Hill, 1984. A brief book that superbly covers the field.

# ANTIPSYCHOTICS 2

## ■ HISTORY

Chlorpromazine was synthesized in 1950. Two years later, Delay and Deniker began to work with it in France. Its effects were so obvious that they knew they had an effective treatment for psychosis after they had treated their first 10 patients. In 1955 this drug began to be used in the United States; largely as a result of the introduction of chlorpromazine, the state hospital population dropped dramatically. Even though the number of people in the United States has doubled, the inpatient census is only one-fourth what it was prior to chlorpromazine. The decreased census is accounted for by a dramatic reduction in the average length of stay, not a drop in the number of admissions. While some of this may be attributed to the community mental health center move-

TABLE 1. **Important Antipsychotics**

| Class/Generic Name | Trade Name | Dose Equivalent (mg) | Comments |
|---|---|---|---|
| **Phenothiazines** | | | |
| Aliphatic | | | |
| Chlorpromazine[a] | Thorazine | 100 | The original antipsychotic, the prototypic low-potency agent. |
| Piperidine | | | |
| Thioridazine[a] | Mellaril | 95 | The only agent with an absolute maximum (800 mg q.d.). This is due to pigmentary retinopathy at higher doses. Very anticholinergic. |
| Mesoridazine | Serentil | 50 | A first-pass metabolite of thioridazine. |
| Piperazine | | | |
| Trifluoperazine[a] | Stelazine | 5 | An early phenothiazine. |
| Fluphenazine[a] | Prolixin<br>Permitil | 2 | Also available as fluphenazine decanoate and enanthate. These are depot forms for which dose equivalents are not available. |
| Dibenzoxazepine | | | |
| Loxapine | Loxitane | 15 | |
| Dihydroindolone | | | |
| Molindone | Lidone<br>Moban | 10 | Possibly associated with weight reduction. |
| Thioxanthenes | | | |
| Thiothixene | Navane | 3 | Has a very high incidence of akathisia. |

| Class/Generic Name | Trade Name | Dose Equivalent (mg) | Comments |
|---|---|---|---|
| Butyrophenone | | | |
| Haloperidol[a] | Haldol | 1.6 | The prototypic high-potency drug. A decanoate form is available. Dose equivalents for it are not available. |
| Dibenzodiazepine | | | |
| Clozapine | | | Not yet available in the United States. Has minimal effects on the $D_2$ receptor, leading to questions about mechanism of action. Minimal extrapyramidal syndromes. High affinity for $alpha_2$, muscarinic, and $histamine_1$ receptors. Very sedating. A high incidence of agranulocytosis in Finland has slowed approval in the United States. |
| Diphenylbutylpiperidine | | | |
| Penfluridol | | | Not yet available in the United States, it is a long-acting (about 1 week) oral agent. Dosage equivalents are unavailable. |
| Pimozide | Orap | | Approved only for Tourette's disorder. |

*Note*. q.d. = per day.
[a] Available generically.

ment of the 1960s, antipsychotics have been the most important factor in emptying the state hospitals.

During the three decades of experience with these drugs there have been cycles in prescribing practices. We have vacillated between high-dose, aggressive treatment and more moderate courses of medication. Increasing awareness of serious toxicity, such as tardive dyskinesia and neuroleptic malignant syndrome, has recently led to a movement back to more temperate use. See Table 1 for a list of important antipsychotics.

## ■ MECHANISM OF ACTION

Unfortunately, there has been little real progress in the basic pharmacology of this area since the introduction of chlorpromazine. With the possible exception of clozapine, all antipsychotics appear to act by blocking the postsynaptic dopamine receptor. Dopamine depletors, such as Rauwolfia alkaloids (e.g., reserpine), also have antipsychotic efficacy, but toxicity limits their use. Progress has been limited to the development of longer acting depot drugs designed to enhance compliance and agents of varying potency with slightly differing toxicities.

The antipsychotics can be seen as occupying a continuum from high to low potency. This is another way of saying that it takes more milligrams of chlorpromazine than haloperidol to have the same effect. Table 1 includes a heading for equivalent doses that can be used as a guide for ordering the drugs this way. Low-potency drugs, such as chlorpromazine, are more sedating, cause more orthostasis, are more likely to have anticholinergic effects, and probably are associated with greater lowering of the seizure threshold than high-potency agents, which are more likely to be associated with extrapyramidal syndromes and neuroleptic malignant syndrome.

Since all antipsychotics act by blocking the dopamine receptor, it follows that they all have similar efficacy if given in equivalent doses. Antipsychotics block other receptors as well. Some of the other effects are listed in Table 2. The varying effect upon histamine$_1$ ($H_1$), alpha, and muscarinic receptors goes a long way toward predicting toxicity.

Understanding these principles makes it clear why *two antipsychotics should never be coprescribed.* Toxicity is additive, but

TABLE 2. **Receptor Affinities of Antipsychotics**

| Drug | $D_2$ Affinity | Standardized $H_1$ Affinity | Standardized $Alpha_1$ Affinity | Standardized Muscarinic Affinity |
|---|---|---|---|---|
| Chlorpromazine | 1 | 1 | 3 | 1 |
| Thioridazine | 1 | 1 | 3 | 3 |
| Mesoridazine | 1 | 3 | 3 | 2 |
| Loxapine | 1 | 3 | 2 | 2 |
| Molindone | 0/1 | 0/1 | 0/1 | 2 |
| Trifluoperazine | 2 | 0/1 | 0/1 | 0/1 |
| Fluphenazine | 4 | 0/1 | 0/1 | 0/1 |
| Thiothixene | 4 | 0/1 | 0/1 | 0/1 |
| Haloperidol | 3 | 0/1 | 1 | 0/1 |
| Clozapine | 0/1 | 4 | 4 | 4 |

*Note.* Data are based on in vitro receptor binding assays with human brain tissue. Standardized affinity = affinity for the given receptor ÷ $D_2$ affinity. 0 = no effect, 4 = market effect. Adapted from Black JL, Richelson E: Antipsychotic drugs: prediction of side-effect profiles based on neuroreceptor data derived from human brain tissue. Mayo Clin Proc 1987; 62:369-372.

the desired effect—blockade of the $dopamine_2$ ($D_2$) receptor is no greater when two drugs are used than it would be when higher doses of one compound are taken.

## ■ INDICATIONS

Antipsychotics, like other psychotropics, treat symptoms, not diseases. These drugs are highly effective in treating agitation, assaultiveness, hallucinations, delusions, and psychomotor excitement arising from a wide variety of etiologies. They are not, however, antischizophrenic or antimanic per se. What follows is a discussion of some of the leading indications grouped by diagnostic category. Even though they are ordered this way, it should be remembered that they treat signs and symptoms, not diagnoses.

### *SCHIZOPHRENIA, SCHIZOPHRENIFORM DISORDER, AND BRIEF REACTIVE PSYCHOSES*

The overwhelming majority of antipsychotic drugs are prescribed for patients with schizophrenia. Review of the target symptoms mentioned above indicates that the medications are quite effective in treating the positive symptoms of schizophrenia but are relatively ineffective at addressing the important negative symptoms of the disorder, such as impaired judgment and insight, amotivation, and flattened affect. These target symptoms do respond at times, albeit slowly, so it is generally worth attempting to address these issues pharmacologically, though they often are most responsive to social skills training and supportive and educational psychotherapy.

### ACUTE PHASE

Several years ago there was enthusiasm for very aggressive initial treatment of thought disorders. This was variously termed *psychotolysis*, *psychiatric digitalizaton*, or *rapid neuroleptization*. Psychotic patients were given 5 to 10 mg of haloperidol intramuscularly (IM) every 30 to 60 minutes until their psychosis cleared. This approach was remarkably well tolerated, but we subsequently learned that the outcome measured a week or more later was no better than that of more moderate treatment. There is still room for this sort of treatment, but it should be reserved for the truly dangerous patient who poses a substantial risk of harm to self or others. This is probably most appropriately termed *rapid tranquilization*, for it assists behavioral control acutely but will probably not treat the underlying delusions, hallucinations, or conceptual disorganization in the long range (1).

Rapid tranquilization involves a relatively simple technique: Haloperidol 5 mg IM can be given acutely, followed by 10 mg orally (p.o.) every (q.) 30 minutes until behavioral control (usually sedation) is realized. If patients reject the oral form, then 5 mg IM can be substituted. It is highly unusual for more than three doses to be required; no more than five should be given. While the initial dose of this regimen is parenteral, subsequent doses should be offered orally. The rationale is that parenteral administration is slightly more rapid in onset, but the difference is not so great as to require continuous intramuscular use. In cases where an even more rapidly acting agent is required, droperidol 5 to 10 mg can be utilized. Droperidol is a butyrophenone, closely related to haloperidol, that is used as an anesthetic agent because of its very rapid onset. It is only available in parenteral form. No more than three doses should be given. Any of these approaches should be regarded as akin to the management of alcohol withdrawal or diabetic ketoacidosis; treatment is keyed around continuous evaluation. There can be no absolute guidelines as to dosing. It should, instead, be a matter of frequent reevaluation and titration.

Recently, in an attempt to minimize antipsychotic exposure, there has been interest in combining neuroleptics with benzodiazepines (BZDs). Lorazepam 1 to 2 mg IM is most frequently used since it is the only BZD with dependable parenteral absorption. The theory is that the BZD will offer sedation during the initial phases of managing an agitated patient. Once more effective antipsychotic control is obtained, the BZD can be phased out (2). While this approach has considerable theoretical appeal, it has not yet been validated in a prospective, placebo-controlled trial.

In the usual nonemergent situation, use a slower, more thoughtful approach. The first steps should involve obtaining a good history and thinking about differential diagnosis. The cornerstones of this manner of thinking are outlined in Chapter 1. Once the history is obtained, the diagnosis reasonably defined, baseline unmedicated behaviors noted, and realistic target behaviors plotted, then initial pharmacotherapy can be attempted. Use of a standardized rating instrument such as the Brief Psychiatric Rating Scale at baseline and weekly thereafter is a useful, reproducible way to document the impact of treatment.

## INITIAL NONACUTE MANAGEMENT

The goal now switches from behavioral control to treatment of more fundamental defects. The aim of pharmacotherapy should now be the treatment of hallucinations, delusions, sleep alterations, mannerisms, stereotypies, and disorders of communication. Negative symptoms such as lack of motivation, difficulty with initiating activities, and diminished insight, judgment, and affect respond more rarely, but are legitimate behaviors to attempt to treat nonetheless.

Selection of the appropriate antipsychotic should depend on which toxicities the particular patient will tolerate best. A recently catatonic patient should not ordinarily receive a high-potency agent for fear of inducing a dystonia that might be misinterpreted. Another patient with concerns about his masculinity would do better with a high-potency agent, thereby minimizing the chance of erectile dysfunction. Remember to pay attention to whatever did or did not work pharmacologically with previous episodes. Past experience is always the best predictor of response.

Selection of an initial dose should depend on size, level of agitation, degree of psychosis, etc. Normative initial daily doses are approximately 5 mg of haloperidol, 200 to 300 mg of chlorpromazine, or the equivalent dose of another antipsychotic agent. The dose can be increased every three to five days, but the practitioner must realize that it may take as long as six weeks for an antipsychotic to take effect. There are no data to establish that doses much beyond 20 mg per day of haloperidol offer any increased benefit. For several of the high-potency drugs there is a strong suggestion that there is a "therapeutic window" or a curvilinear dose–response curve. With such a drug, a dose that is too high is every bit as ineffective as one that is too low. The difficult part of this phase of treatment is resisting the pressure to move too quickly. The urgency will come from the physician, from the patient, and from concerned staff, all of whom will sense the patient's pain and want immediate intervention to end it. Unfortunately, there seems to be a certain time frame that cannot be accelerated. Overly vigorous initial treatment may expose the patient to drugs that are not necessary and may even retard progress.

## THE TREATMENT-REFRACTORY PATIENT

Patients refractory to conventional treatment during the initial phase pose a special challenge. When patients fail to respond to six weeks of a moderate dose of an antipsychotic, a series of questions should be asked:

1. Is the patient correctly diagnosed? Failure to respond to conventional treatment should always lead to diagnostic doubt. The possibilities could include a major depression with psychotic features, drug toxicity, a primary neurologic disorder, etc.

2. Is the patient in fact taking the medication? It is difficult to overestimate the extent of noncompliance.
3. Is the patient absorbing the drug appropriately? Eventually the measurement of antipsychotic drug levels may be an indication of how much of a neuroleptic a patient is absorbing, but interpretation of the assay is currently so unsophisticated as to tell us only if *any* drug is to be found in blood. As such there is little indication for these assays in the presence of any side effects, since we can determine that the patient is getting at least some effect from the drug. Commercial laboratories will quote "therapeutic" levels for these tests, but there is, at best, a very crude correlation between blood level and response. Keep in mind that any treatment plan that hinges on a blood level for an antipsychotic is premature.

   One does, on occasion, see patients who respond to depot, injectable antipsychotics but not to oral agents. It is not clear whether this represents a form of malabsorption, enhanced compliance, or some other phenomenon, but use of a parenteral agent can provide a legitimate alternative for the patient who has not responded to an oral medication. The possibility that a patient is an outlier who requires higher than normal doses of medication should always be seriously considered before switching to another compound. In the absence of toxicity an increase of dose should be one of the first steps in treating the refractory patient.
4. Is the patient unresponsive to one antipsychotic but a candidate for another? One rarely sees patients who fail to respond to one compound but respond quite well to another. Usually it is wisest to switch to a completely new class of drugs (for example, to switch from a phenothiazine to a butyrophenone or a dihydroindolone).

   If a patient has failed to respond to several antipsychotics, including oral and parenteral forms, then there are other possibilities to be considered. Lithium or carbamazepine in combination with antipsychotics can offer additional benefit beyond what can be offered by the antipsychotic alone. This is discussed further in Chapter 4.

Electroconvulsive therapy is an alternative to drug therapy that can help some schizophrenic patients (see Chapter 5).

Megadose antipsychotics have never been shown to be of benefit in controlled trials, but individual patients clearly have benefited, and daily doses as high as 1200 mg of fluphenazine HCl seem remarkably well tolerated (3).

One should not overlook nonbiological treatments. Behavioral and family treatments can be quite effective. Insight-oriented techniques should probably still be viewed as experimental with this population, but can be of significant benefit to certain individuals.

There are no scientific data to support the use of megavitamins, beta-blockers, dialysis, or psychosurgery. Each has had its vogue, but has passed from the scene. The danger of such approaches is that they hold out a false promise to patients and their families.

## MAINTENANCE TREATMENT

The aims now are to maintain the gains of the initial phase, perhaps even furthering them, and to prevent the return of acute illness. Once again, biologic treatment should be integrated into a broader program including psychological, occupational, and family interventions.

How long to maintain a patient on pharmacotherapy is the art, rather than the science, of psychopharmacology. Frequent, severe prior episodes that occurred without much of a prodrome would be persuasive arguments for more prolonged maintenance. The presence of insight into the developing illness is vital if a patient's medication is to be safely discontinued. A strong family history of schizophrenia and poor premorbid functioning increase the likelihood that medicine will need to be maintained. The quality of your relationship with the patient and his family is a very important part of the decision making. A trusting relationship will give you access to the data needed to assess

1. How likely the patient is to deteriorate,
2. How much warning there will be,
3. How difficult a decompensation would be to bring under control, and
4. How likely the patient would be to seek help.

When maintenance neuroleptics are discontinued they should be slowly tapered. Antipsychotics are highly lipophilic drugs that, as a result, take a long time to be cleared from the body. It is not unusual for a patient to decompensate several months after stopping medication. Typically, the patient fails to make an association between the suspension of the medicine and the psychotic break; compliance is therefore not fostered. This long latency between discontinuing medication and the resulting decompensation should encourage a very slow, gradual taper of the medication over the course of several months. There are three possible outcomes:

1. Decompensation may occur rapidly, indicating the need for resumption of the full dose of medication;
2. Breakthrough of some symptoms may occur, indicating that an intermediate dose should be maintained; or
3. The patient may do very well, indicating that no medicine is necessary.

Maintenance with antipsychotics should probably be reserved for schizophrenic patients; the risk of tardive dyskinesia is higher for patients with affective disorders, and there are few other indications for prolonged treatment.

## *MANIA*

Both lithium and carbamazepine work well acutely for mania. Antipsychotics simply make the response somewhat more rapid. If used, they should be for the short term only, with prophylaxis offered by one of the thymopleptics. The possibility of substituting benzodiazepines for some or all of a neuroleptic regimen during an acute manic episode is being explored, but is not yet well supported.

## *PSYCHOTIC DEPRESSION*

Ranking of efficacy is as follows:

1. Electroconvulsive therapy
2. Combination of an antipsychotic and an antidepressant

3. An antidepressant alone
4. An antipsychotic alone

Once again, it should be emphasized that patients generally should not be maintained on antipsychotics, since antidepressants usually will do an effective job without exposing patients to the risk of tardive dyskinesia.

## *DEMENTIA AND DELIRIUM*

Antipsychotics have long been used to treat agitation in demented patients. They will, at times, be helpful, but it should be realized that treatment is largely empirical. The few good, controlled trials available suggest that high-potency agents are preferred and that, as with schizophrenia, they are helpful with agitation, assaultiveness, hyperactivity, and hallucinations, but not with apathy or withdrawal (4). The significant anticholinergic impact of low-potency antipsychotics in cognitively compromised patients means that high-potency agents should be used except with patients who are already parkinsonian. The initial dose should be approximately one-third to one-fifth of that used with younger patients. An adequate trial should last at least one month. In delirium, brief use of an antipsychotic may be helpful in obtaining behavioral control while the primary cause is addressed. Similar strategy to that described in the section on acute management is appropriate.

## *ANXIETY*

Antipsychotics are reasonably efficacious anxiolytics, but they should not be used as such given their toxicity and the availability of alternative agents and approaches.

## *TOURETTE'S DISORDER*

Haloperidol 0.5 to 5 mg daily (q.d.) is helpful with both the motor and vocal tics of Tourette's disorder. Pimozide has been approved by the FDA only for the treatment of this disorder. Doses usually range from 6 to 20 mg q.d. Higher doses have been associated with bradycardia and QT prolongation on the electrocardiogram, so this drug should probably be reserved for patients who are either unresponsive to haloperidol or experiencing problems with it. Clonidine has also been of benefit and may have less potential toxicity. Hypotension often limits how much can be given, and the desired effects of the drug may not be seen for several months. Typical doses may range from 0.15 to 0.60 mg q.d.

## ■ SIDE EFFECTS

### *COMMON, EARLY SIDE EFFECTS*

By virtue of their blockade of the dopamine receptor, antipsychotics can cause signs and symptoms that so closely mimic idiopathic parkinsonism as to be indistinguishable from it. These extrapyramidal syndromes (EPS), which include dystonias, parkinsonism, and akathisia, are more likely to occur with high-potency antipsychotics, may wax and wane, will disappear with sleep, and may increase with emotional stress. The likelihood of a drug's inducing EPS correlates highly with its ability to block the dopamine receptor.

*Acute dystonias* classically occur within one to five days of the initiation of treatment or with an increase in dose. Common presentations include opisthotonus, torticollis, and oculogyric crises, but almost any part of the body can be involved. Rarely, laryngeal involvement can occur, at times being so severe as to require intubation. These are most common with young males. These reactions are extremely frightening to an unprepared patient, so all young males, especially outpatients, should be forewarned about this possibility and encouraged to seek prompt treatment. Treatment is with diphenhydramine 25–50 mg or benzotropine 1 to 2 mg intravenously (IV). Patients will respond within minutes.

*Drug-induced parkinsonism* presents with all of the usual signs, including masked facies, cogwheeling, three-cyele-per-second tremor, festinant gait, stiffness, and drooling. Peak risk appears between 5 and 75 days after initiating treatment or after increasing the dose. Routine use of a standardized exam to monitor EPS is encouraged. A slightly modified version of a commonly used exam is included below in Table 3. Treatment for any of the EPS is to decrease the dose, to switch to a lower potency drug, or to treat with one of the agents listed in Table 4. If one of these drugs is used, it should be reviewed within several weeks to months, since they generally can be withdrawn. All too often, once prescribed, antiparkinsonians are routinely maintained, exposing patients to needless expense and toxicity.

All of the antiparkinsonians listed have short half-lives and should be prescribed on a twice daily (b.i.d.) or thrice daily (t.i.d.) basis. The half-lives of antipsychotics are much longer. Anticholinergics and related compounds should therefore be con-

TABLE 3. **Suggested Exam for Extrapyramidal Syndromes**

1. Observe gait, paying particular attention to arm swing, and posture.
   0 = normal; 1 = decreased arm swing; 2 = No. 1 plus obvious rigidity; 3 = stiff gait, arms rigid before abdomen; 4 = stooped, shuffling with propulsion and retropulsion.
2. You and the patient should stand with arms extended to the side at shoulder height. On a signal let them drop.
   0 = normal with loud slap and rebound as they hit the side of the body; 1 = slowed drop, little rebound; 2 = no rebound; 3 = markedly slowed, no slap; 4 = arms fall very slowly as if against resistance.
3. Rotate elbow and monitor the wrist with your other hand. Rate both arms separately for stiffness and cogwheeling. The same procedures can be done for the legs. Rate on a 0–4 basis.
4. Have patient hold out hands. Observe tremor then and at rest.
   0 = normal; 1 = mild finger tremor; 2 = tremor of finger and hands; 3 = limb tremor; 4 = whole body tremor.
5. Have patient open his or her mouth and raise his or her tongue to assess salivation.
   0 = normal; 1 = pooling with maneuvers above; 2 = occasional problems with speech due to drooling; 3 = as with 2, but frequent; 4 = frank drooling.
6. You and the patient should place your hands on a table. Begin to tap your index finger as rapidly as possible. Repeat with both hands. Monitor for bradykinesia.
   0 = normal; 1 = mild slowing; 2 = moderate slowing; 3 = severe slowing; 4 = virtually immobilized.

Modified from Simpson GM, Angus JWJ: A rating scale for extrapyramidal side effects. Acta Psychiatr Scand 1970; 212 Supp: 11-19.

tinued for several days after the discontinuation of an antipsychotic. Anticholinergics are not without their own toxicity. The mnemonic about atropine should be remembered: "dry as a bone, red as a beet, blind as a bat, mad as a hatter." Constipation, visual blurring, erectile dysfunction, and urinary retention, especially in patients with enlarged prostates, should be added to the litany of potential problems associated with anticholinergic effects. Amantadine differs in that it is a dopamine agonist. It is significantly more expensive and there is a question as to whether its effectiveness is maintained over the long haul, but it does provide an alternative to anticholinergic toxicity in vulnerable patients. It should also be remembered that low-potency agents, especially thioridazine, mesoridazine, and clozapine, are potent anticholinergics in their own right. Combination of these drugs with

TABLE 4. **Agents for the Treatment of Extrapyramidal Syndromes**

| Class/Generic Name | Trade Name | Usual Dose | Comments |
|---|---|---|---|
| Anticholinergics | | | |
| Benztropine[a] | Cogentin | 0.5–2 mg t.i.d. | 1–2 mg intravenously (IV) for acute dystonia |
| Biperiden | Akineton | 2 mg o.d.–t.i.d. | |
| Procyclidine | Kemadrin | 2.5–7.5 mg t.i.d. | |
| Trihexyphenidyl[a] | Artane | 1–5 mg t.i.d. | 2 mg IV for acute dystonia |
| Antihistamines | | | |
| Diphenhydramine[a] | Benadryl | 12.5–50 mg t.i.d. or q.i.d. | 25–50 mg IV for acute dystonia |
| Beta-blockers | | | |
| Propranolol[a] | Inderal and others | 10–20 mg q.i.d. | For akathisia, but not other extrapyramidal syndromes |

*Note.* t.i.d. = three times a day; q.i.d. = four times a day.
[a] Available generically.

other anticholinergic agents, including many tricyclics such as amitriptyline, can leave a patient vulnerable to delirium.

*Akathisia* differs from other forms of EPS. It is a purely sensory phenomenon, typically presenting as a poorly described sense of restlessness, usually felt most strongly in the legs, which causes people to pace. Patients may have difficulty remaining seated throughout an interview and will frequently shift about, crossing and uncrossing their legs. Unlike other forms of EPS, tolerance rarely develops to this symptom. The period of maximal risk is from 5 to 60 days after exposure. Frequently this is misdiagnosed as agitation, leading to an increase in the antipsychotic, when what is needed is a decrease, a switch to a lower potency agent, or treatment with an anticholinergic or a beta-blocker. Compared to the other forms of EPS, akathisia is the least likely to respond to antiparkinsonians. A trail may well be warranted nonetheless. Alternatively, treatment with propranolol 20 to 60 mg q.d., or the equivalent with another lipophilic centrally acting beta-blocker, seems to work quite well (5).

*Akinesia* is one of the more subtle forms of toxicity that antipsychotics can induce. It is characterized by diminished spontaneity with decreased speech, few gestures, apathy, and indifference. There is often a difficult three-way differential among drug-induced akinesia, postpsychotic depression, and undertreated schizophrenia with negative symptoms predominating. Here a careful history should help. If signs and symptoms are caused by undertreatment, then the symptoms should have been present all along. If they are present secondary to postpsychotic depression, then depressive cognition should be present. If the cause is the drug, then the symptoms should be dose dependent. In this case, they should be treated like any other EPS. Some clinicians argue that this is so ubiquitous and so difficult to diagnose that routine prophylactic antiparkinsonian treatment is required. Antiparkinsonian agents should not be reflexively used, but one should maintain a high index of suspicion and a low threshold for antiparkinsonian use.

*Sedation* is common with low-potency agents. At times this may be desired; at other times it is not. The patient frequently accommodates to sedation over time. This symptom correlates with antihistaminic effects.

*Orthostatic hypotension* correlates with a drug's blockade of the alpha receptor. Low-potency drugs are more likely to do this. This may be a dose-limiting factor, particularly with the elderly. In measuring orthostasis it is best to measure blood pressure and pulse while the patient is sitting or lying, after standing, and again while still standing five minutes later. This should be correlated with a patient's complaints of lightheadedness or dizziness. Patients should be warned of this possibility and encouraged to get up slowly from prolonged lying or sitting.

*Anticholinergic side effects* can be problematic for those drugs with high standardized muscarinic affinity. These may include urinary retention, especially in patients with enlarged prostates; erectile and ejaculatory disturbances; visual blurring; and dry mouth. The dry mouth and the blurred vision frequently improve with time.

## *TARDIVE DYSKINESIA*

Tardive dyskinesia (TD) has become an increasing source of concern. It is defined as abnormal, stereotypic, involuntary movements caused by exposure to prolonged dopamine blockade, as with antipsychotics. It is thought that the receptor compensates by up-regulating or increasing the number of dopamine receptors and also increasing the avidity with which the receptor seeks the transmitter.

While buccolingual movements are the most common, any muscle, including even the diaphragm, can be involved. Movements are classically choreoathetotic, but may involve tremor or more static posturing even to the point of dystonia. The movements disappear during sleep. Patients may be able to suppress them briefly. They will increase with stress. Movement elsewhere in the body, as with distracting maneuvers such as finger tapping, will increase the dyskinesia. The movements will initially get worse as the antipsychotic is withdrawn, but this is clearly the appropriate long-range strategy. Although increasing the dose will lead to short-term improvement as the up-regulated receptors are blocked, the gain will be but temporary as new receptors will begin to sprout. Thus the temporary solution afforded by increasing the dose of the antipsychotic will ultimately only escalate the problem.

## DIFFERENTIAL DIAGNOSIS

The differential is long and complicated. Extrapyramidal syndromes can, at times, be difficult to distinguish from TD. Decreasing the dose of the antipsychotic can help because EPS should improve and TD should initially worsen. Schizophrenic patients postured and had involuntary movements long before antipsychotics were introduced. Finding unmedicated schizophrenic patients is difficult, but recent studies show chronic, unmedicated patients as evincing serious involuntary movements. It is further estimated that 5% of normal geriatric patients will have idiopathic senescent dyskinesias. Patients on neuroleptics may show involuntary movements when their drugs are abruptly withdrawn. This is termed *withdrawal dyskinesia* and may represent one of the earliest manifestations of the disorder. There are conflicting data as to whether periodic withdrawal is helpful or harmful. Animal models suggest that periodic discontinuation may create more problems, but drug holidays clearly have diagnostic value because withdrawal dyskinesia should alert the physician to make every attempt possible to stop the medication.

All patients should be routinely monitored with a reliable rating instrument. The Abnormal Involuntary Movement Scale (AIMS) is the most widely used and is as good as any (see Table 5). It can be filled out as you interview patients. With practice it can be completed in several minutes.

Disagreement as to diagnostic criteria accounts for some of the wide variability in the estimates of TD's incidence and prevalence, but the incidence is probably about 15% (6). It is similarly problematic to define the percentage of patients who will reverse with discontinuation of the drug. Probably between one-third and one-half of dyskinetic patients will not reverse even if made drug free. This is a frightening statistic that should make us reserve antipsychotics for patients who truly need them.

## RISK FACTORS

Certain risk factors should make us particularly circumspect. Elderly patients are less likely to reverse upon discontinuation. Patients with affective disorders get far worse TD and at an earlier age than do their schizophrenic congeners. One should not lose track of the tremendous good that neuroleptics can do, but they should be reserved for those patients who really need them. Intuitively it makes sense to prescribe antipsychotics at the lowest possible dose, but neither length of exposure, total exposure, use of anticholinergics, nor maximum dose have been documented as risk factors.

TABLE 5. **Abnormal Involuntary Movement Scale**

1. Observe gait on the way into the room.
2. Have patient remove gum or dentures if ill fitting.
3. See is the patient is aware of any movements.
4. Have the patient sit on a firm chair without arms with his hands on his knees, legs slightly apart, and feet flat on the floor. Now and throughout the exam, look at the entire body for movements.
5. Have the patient sit with hands unsupported, dangling over the knees.
6. Ask patient to open his mouth twice. Look for tongue movements.
7. Ask patient to protrude his tongue twice.
8. Ask patient to tap thumb against each finger for 15 seconds with each hand. Observe face and legs.
9. Have patient stand with arms extended forward.

Rate each item on a 0–4 scale for the highest severity observed. Movements that occur only upon activation merit one point less than those which occur spontaneously.

0 = none; 1 = minimal, may be extreme normal; 2 = mild; 3 = moderate; 4 = severe

| | | | | | | |
|---|---|---|---|---|---|---|
| Facial and Oral Movements: | 1. Muscles of Facial Expression | 0 | 1 | 2 | 3 | 4 |
| | 2. Lips and Perioral Area | 0 | 1 | 2 | 3 | 4 |
| | 3. Jaw | 0 | 1 | 2 | 3 | 4 |
| | 4. Tongue | 0 | 1 | 2 | 3 | 4 |
| Extremity Movements: | 5. Upper | 0 | 1 | 2 | 3 | 4 |
| | 6. Lower | 0 | 1 | 2 | 3 | 4 |
| Trunk Movements: | 7. Neck, shoulders, hips | 0 | 1 | 2 | 3 | 4 |
| Global Judgments: | 8. Severity of abnormal movements | 0 | 1 | 2 | 3 | 4 |
| | 9. Incapacitation due to abnormal movements | 0 | 1 | 2 | 3 | 4 |
| | 10. Patient's awareness of abnormal movements<br>0 = Unaware  4 = Severe distress | 0 | 1 | 2 | 3 | 4 |

Modified from Guy W: ECDEU Assessment Manual for Psychopharmacology. Rockville, MD, U.S. Department of Health, Education and Welfare, 1976.

## TREATMENT

There are rather shaky epidemiologic findings indicating that thioridazine may pose less risk. This fits with one pathogenetic theory that states that there is an imbalance between dopaminergic and cholinergic activity and that a maximally anticholinergic drug would pose the least risk.

There is no proven treatment for TD. Any therapy must therefore be regarded as experimental. The cornerstone should be discontinuation of the antipsychotic, but this should not be done reflexively. The decision whether or not to stop the drug presents a profound ethical dilemma. A judgment has to be made as to whether the risk of worsening TD is graver than the risk of worsening psychosis. This is a difficult dilemma and a choice that most therapists prefer not to make alone. Many patients have a kind of agnosia about the movements. They know that they are there because others have commented on them, but they themselves are not terribly concerned. The decision should be made by the patient if competent, and by the family if not, after receiving input from the physician.

## WITHDRAWAL

If drug withdrawal is to be helpful the results are usually apparent within the first three to six months. If the movements continue, and if they are sufficiently severe as to require treatment, then several alternatives can be investigated. Dopamine depleters have the advantage of having some antipsychotic efficacy. Dopamine depletion has not been associated with the onset of TD, although depression and hypotension have been associated with the use of reserpine. Treatment is initiated with 0.25 mg q.d., with similar daily increments, ultimately dividing the dose q.i.d. The maximal dose is about 6 mg q.d. Orthostatic blood pressure should be monitored throughout the trial.

There is a reciprocal antagonism between striatal acetylcholine and dopamine. Increasing acetylcholine should therefore ameliorate TD. Physostigmine, an inhibitor of cholinesterase that degrades acetylcholine, has proved helpful, but it is short acting and has to be given IV. Other cholinergic agonists are either toxic or ineffective. Gamma-aminobutyric acid inhibits nigrostriatal dopamine activity. Benzodiazepines therefore have theoretical appeal, but they have to be used at such high doses as to be of no clinical utility.

In summary then, TD represents a condition that may or may not be reversible and for which there is no effective treatment. It is desirable to discontinue the antipsychotic if possible, but this decision should be reached by the patient and his or her family with input from the physician. The primary intervention should be preventative. Antipsychotics should be reserved for patients who truly need them. An explanation of the possibility of TD should be made as soon as the patient has cleared sufficiently to offer true informed consent. Patients should be regularly assessed with the AIMS or a similar instrument, and periodic drug holidays should be attempted in an attempt to provoke withdrawal dyskinesia.

## *RARER TOXICITIES*

Low-potency agents, such as chlorpromazine or thioridazine in particular, are thought to *lower the seizure threshold*. This belief is based on little hard data, but it is probably prudent to use a high-potency agent, like haloperidol, in patients with history of seizure disorder, and they should not be used with patients who are withdrawing from central nervous system (CNS) depressants.

High-dose, low-potency drugs, particularly in young males, have been associated with *drug-induced catatonia*. If this is the case, then the patient should improve if the drug is withdrawn or if an anticholinergic is added.

Antipsychotics *prolong ventricular repolarization*. Thioridazine is the most offensive, but this is generally more a theoretical than a real problem. They also may be associated with an increased QR interval and T-wave flattening.

*Retrograde ejaculation* can occur with thioridazine. *Increased appetite* and *weight gain* are not unusual. Molindone, for some reason, seems immune from this effect. *Galactorrhea* and *gynecomastia* can occur. They are associated with an increase in the prolactin level. Dopamine is thought to be prolactin-releasing inhibitory factor, so it is not surprising that prolactin levels increase and these effects eventuate. *Menstrual irregularities* are not infrequent. Patients should be warned that these medicines are not a reliable form of birth control.

Phenothiazines in particular have been associated with *hepatitis*. Liver biopsies show a cholestatic picture. This typically occurs early in the course of treatment. There is little evidence of cross-sensitivity with nonphenothiazine neuroleptics. *Agranulocytosis* has been very rare, typically with low-potency drugs, but patients should have complete blood counts drawn with signs of infection. *Photosensitivity* is common with low potency agents. Patients should be given sunscreens routinely. *Lenticular and corneal deposits* have been reported with phenothiazines. Thioridazine has led to pigmentary retinopathy at doses of 1 g q.d. The FDA has, as a result, imposed a ceiling of 800 mg q.d. Hypothalamic dysfunction may be associated with *poikilothermia*, or a loss of temperature regulation such that there is a tendency toward hyperthermia in the summer and hypothermia in the winter. This is particularly likely in the elderly. The *syndrome of inappropriate antidiuretic hormone* has been reported.

Neuroleptic-induced *supersensitivity psychosis* has been reported by Chouinard. He describes patients who also have tardive dyskinesia and appear to require escalating doses of neuroleptic to maintain the same effect. Missing a single dose or getting to the end of a depot cycle is associated with positive symptoms. This is thought to represent extension of dopaminergic hypersensitivity to the mesolimbic system, in addition to the neostriatal involvement associated with tardive dyskinesia (7).

*Neuroleptic malignant syndrome* (NMS) is a potentially lethal reaction to antipsychotics characterized by muscular rigidity, decreased level of consciousness, and autonomic dysfunction including hyperthermia, labile blood pressure, tachycardia, and diaphoresis. Laboratory findings include elevated creatinine phosphokinase and leukocytosis. It can occur either early or late in the course of neuroleptic treatment and is far more common with high-potency drugs. Coprescription of lithium appears to be a risk factor. It has also been seen after the withdrawal of dopamine agonists. The differential is quite complicated. A clinically indistinguishable syndrome (Bell's Mania) was described more than a hundred years before the first antipsychotic. Patients need to have a full workup for a fever of unknown origin. The fatality rate is approximately 15%. Various treatments have been suggested, including bromocriptine, amantadine, and dantrolene.

While it is not definite that aggressive treatment is helpful, it is certain that antipsychotics need to be discontinued and that supportive treatment with antipyretics, antihypertensives, antiarrythmics, and whatever other agents are necessary needs to be instituted (8). If rhabdomyolysis leads to renal failure, then dialysis may be necessary. Low-dose heparin may prevent pulmonary emboli in the NMS patient who may be immobilized. Dantrolene inhibits the release of intracellular calcium, thereby preventing heat generated by tonic muscular contraction. This has led to its use in malignant hyperthermia. It is used in doses of 0.8–2.5 mg/kg q. six hours in the patient with NMS. Alternatively, dopamine agonists (amantadine 100 mg b.i.d. or bromocriptine 2.5–20 mg t.i.d.) are used on the basis of the theory that reduced dopaminergic function is the cause of NMS. Many patients who have had such treatments have improved, but some have died, and it is not clear that they alter the natural course of the disor-

TABLE 6. **Antipsychotic Interactions**

| Interacting Agent | Effect | Comments |
|---|---|---|
| Alcohol | Additive effect | Patients should be told that one drink may seem like several |
| Barbiturates | Increase neuroleptic metabolism | |
| Beta-blockers | Risk of orthostasis | |
| Bethanidine, Guanadrel, Guanethedine | Decreased antihypertensive effect | Uptake is blocked |
| Levodopa | Decreased levodopa effect | Inhibits dopamine uptake |
| Lithium | Increased incidence of NMS epidemiologically | Can be coprescribed, but monitor for NMS |
| Nonsteroidal anti-inflammatory agents | Extreme drowsiness | Reported with haloperidol and indomethacin |

*Note:* NMS = neuroleptic malignant syndrome.

der. Controlled trials are virtually impossible with these patients so treatment will need to continue to be empirical.

## ■ INTERACTIONS

Drug–drug interactions with the neuroleptics are largely predictable from each drug's receptor effects. Those compounds high on the spectrum of muscarinic affinity should not be combined with other anticholinergic agents. Drugs that are potent alpha blockers should be monitored closely if combined with agents that promote orthostasis. Drugs that have significant standardized $H_1$ affinity pose risk for excessive sedation if combined with other CNS depressants. A list of some of the more commonly encountered interactions is presented in Table 6.

## ■ DEPOT ANTIPSYCHOTICS

Most neuroleptics have half-lives of 24 hours or more. Thus they can ordinarily be prescribed each day at bedtime. Sedation is less of a problem and compliance is enhanced by once-daily dosing. Longer acting, or depot, antipsychotics have been developed in an attempt to further ensure adherence to a prescribed regimen.

Currently, there are three depot agents available in the United States (see Table 7). All are given parenterally, but have the advantage of only needing to be given every one to four weeks. Compliance is ensured and there is no worry about absorption. On the other hand, problems may take a long time to correct themselves. The half-lives are so long that it will take a considerable period to reach steady state and a similarly long time to wash out if problems develop.

These medicines are appropriately reserved for patients with malabsorption of oral medication, demonstrated histories of noncompliance, marked ambivalence about medication, or prominent risk factors for drug defaulting, such as ego-syntonic delusional systems. With such patients, long-acting medications can make a dramatic difference. Depot agents are most typically used for the maintenance phase of treatment, but they can be used during the initial, nonacute phase as well. Their toxicities are those that would be expected for any high-potency neuroleptic.

TABLE 7. **Depot Antipsychotic Agents**

| Compound | Dosage/Interval | Approximate Single-Dose Plasma Half-Life (Days) | Approximate Single-Dose Peak Level Obtained (Days) |
|---|---|---|---|
| Fluphenazine decanoate[a] | 12.5–50 mg q. 1–3 weeks | 7 | 1 |
| Fluphenazine enanthate[a] | 12.5–50 mg q. 1–2 weeks | 4 | 2 |
| Haloperidol decanoate | 25–150 mg q. 3–5 weeks | 21 | 7 |

*Note.* q. = every.
[a] Available generically.

Normative doses are 12.5 to 50 mg of fluphenazine decanoate every one to three weeks, or 25 to 150 mg of haloperidol decanoate every three to five weeks. Steady state will not be reached until approximately four times the half-life. Until that time patients previously maintained on oral regimens should continue their oral agent with a gradual taper while the depot level is climbing. The initial dose of the depot agent is difficult to gauge, but the usual factors, including size, age, and degree of psychosis and agitation, should be taken into account. Once an initial, preferably low-dose regimen has been achieved, then both dose and duration will have to be adjusted. The two key questions are whether the peak dose is sufficient to offer antipsychotic effect and whether it is lasting long enough.

## ■ ANTIPSYCHOTICS NOT YET AVAILABLE IN THE UNITED STATES

Penfluridol and fluspirilene are long-acting agents that can be taken orally on a weekly basis. They are approved in Europe and are being tested here.

Clozapine is of great theoretical interest. It is an effective antipsychotic, yet seems to have very little effect on the dopamine receptor and produces minimal EPS. Theoretically it would seem to pose little liability for TD. There were problems in Finland, but not elsewhere, with an epidemic of clozapine-associated agranulocytosis. It is being tested in the United States.

## ■ REFERENCES


1. Dubin WR, Weiss KJ, Dorn JM: Pharmacotherapy of psychiatric emergencies. J Clin Psychopharmacol 1986; 6:210-222
2. Salzman C, Green AI, Rodriguez-Villa F, et al: Benzodiazepines combined with neuroleptics for management of severe disruptive behavior. Psychosomatics 1986; 27, suppl:17-22
3. Linden R, Davis JM, Rubinstern J: High vs. low dose treatment with antipsychotic agents. Psychiatric Annals 1982; 12:769-781
4. Raskind MA, Risse SC, Lampe TH: Dementia and antipsychotic drugs. J Clin Psychiatry 1987; 48(5, suppl):16-18
5. DuPuis B, Catteau J, Dumon JP, et al: Comparison of propranolol, sotalol, and betaxolol in the treatment of neuroleptic-induced akathisia. Am J Psychiatry 1987; 144:802-805
6. Kane JM, Smith JM: Tardive dyskinesia: prevalence and risk factors. Arch Gen Psychiatry 1982; 39:473-481
7. Chouinard G, Jones BD: Neuroleptic-induced supersensitivity psychosis: clinical and pharmacological characteristics. Am J Psychiatry 1980; 137:16-21
8. Levenson JL: Neuroleptic malignant syndrome. Am J Psychiatry 1985; 142:1137-1145


# 3 ANTIDEPRESSANTS

## ■ HISTORY

By 1953 there were suggestions that iproniazid, a monoamine oxidase inhibitor (MAOI) used for the treatment of tuberculosis, had antidepressant properties. Until then, stimulants and electroconvulsive therapy (ECT) were the only biological treatments for depression. Further progress was made with the discovery of imipramine in 1957: The effects were so clear that Roland Kuhn knew he had an important new agent by the time that the third patient had taken the drug. Since chlorpromazine was discovered at approximately the same time, there was great hope for a pharmacological cure of mental illness. We remain considerably short of that goal, but there is little question that antidepressants are a very significant addition.

## ■ TARGET SYMPTOMS

In Chapter 1 it was emphasized that antidepressants do not treat depression, but rather the vegetative signs associated with the syndrome. Table 1 highlights the distinction between the targets for psychotherapy and for the biological therapy of depression. The important point is that the two treatments are additive (1). Medication will help with the hopelessness and anergia that make psychological interventions virtually impossible with a deeply depressed patient. A solid relationship with a patient will, in turn, reinforce medication compliance and increase the likelihood of having sufficient information to make rational pharmacological choices.

The vegetative signs include sleep interruption, particularly early morning awakening; anorexia with weight loss; constipation; psychomotor changes; diurnal variation (with mood worse in the morning); and diminished libido. It should be noted that this reasonably approximates the *Diagnostic and Statistical Manual of Mental Disorders, Third Edition, Revised (DSM-III-R)* definition of melancholia (2). Symptoms such as guilt, anhedonia (absence of pleasure), anergia (diminished energy), hopelessness,

TABLE 1. **Effects of Psychotherapy and Somatic Therapy in Depression**

| Therapy | Signs and Symptoms Relieved | Time Course |
|---|---|---|
| Psychotherapy | Mood, suicide ideation, work, interests, guilt, social adjustment | 4-8 weeks |
| Somatic therapy | Vegetative symptoms, especially sleep and appetite disturbance | 1–3 weeks |

From DiMascio A, Weissman MM, Prosoff BA, et al: Differential symptom reduction by drugs and psychotherapy depression. Arch Gen Psychiatry 1979; 36:1450-1456.

and helplessness may also respond to antidepressants but are not as robust predictors of good outcome.

The typical, but not invariable, pattern of improvement is for signs to respond before symptoms. Patients should be forewarned about this since this information may encourage them to remain in treatment. Others will notice a change before the patient is aware of it; humor may return before mood, sleep may normalize several days before guilt feelings diminish. Many toxicities are immediate, whereas the antidepressant effect often takes several weeks. Seriously depressed patients are also often imbued with a profound sense of hopelessness that leaves them certain that nothing can help. Unless directly addressed, these issues often result in drug defaulters.

## ■ CONTRAINDICATIONS

One must always rule out the "organic" causes of depression; that is, depression secondary to other disease processes. Any good basic psychiatry text will furnish you with a long list of illnesses and toxicities to be considered. A less than exhaustive discussion of some of the more common etiologies follows.

Always consider the possibility of a toxic reaction to medication or other exogenous substance. The key step is to review medication and drug intake in an attempt to correlate them with the onset of the depression. Reserpine, clonidine, and methyldopa are often associated with depression; lipophilic beta-blockers may well be. Central nervous system (CNS) depressants, notably barbiturates and benzodiazepines, are potential offenders as well. Withdrawal from stimulants can be problematic.

Carcinoma of any type, but especially of the pancreas, can present with depression. Dementia, irrespective of etiology, can manifest depression prior to overt cognitive impairment. Almost any systemic infection can do this as well.

A wide variety of metabolic and endocrine disorders can result in the syndrome. Thyroid abnormality, especially hypothyroidism, is frequently associated with depression. The same can be said for adrenal dysfunction, hyperparathyroidism, diabetes, and $B_{12}$ and folate deficiencies. These illnesses serve to underscore the importance of a good review of systems.

It should be remembered that sadness is not the same as

depression. It is, instead, one feature of a syndrome; some cases may lack depressed mood and instead present with irritability. By the same token, the presence of a significant stressor should not necessarily dissuade you from using an antidepressant (see the discussion of adjustment disorder with depressed mood).

Caution should be exercised in patients with history of mania either in themselves or in family members. Any antidepressant treatment has the potential of cycling a depressed patient into mania. Patients with significant risk factors should probably have lithium prophylaxis along with the antidepressant.

The medical contraindications are primarily cardiac and are discussed in the section on toxicity.

## ■ INDICATIONS

### *DEPRESSION*

#### MAJOR DEPRESSION, RECURRENT OR SINGLE EPISODE

The vegetative signs previously discussed remain the most important predictors of response. The efficacy of antidepressants in this disorder is clear. The usual figures quoted are that 50% of patients will resolve within six weeks with no treatment, 55% with placebo, 65% with an MAOI, 70% with a heterocyclic antidepressant (HCA), and 85 to 90% with ECT. Many believe that the response percentages quoted for active treatment are low and are much better if thorough and aggressive therapy is provided. The figures would also improve if the studies were limited to patients with melancholia. Other positive predictors are intuitively obvious: past personal or even family history of response to medication, and good premorbid or intermorbid functioning. The impressive response to no treatment or placebo serves to remind us that acute depression is often a self-limiting illness and that medications will, at times, do no more than accelerate the resolution of the process.

Some common errors to avoid:

1. Thinking that a little bit of depression merits a little bit of drug. If you are going to treat, then nothing less than a full therapeutic dose should be used. To do otherwise

merely exposes the patient to toxicity without the opportunity for benefit.

2. Not treating for a long enough period. All antidepressant treatments take two to three weeks to work. Unfortunately, this process cannot be accelerated. Do not give up on an agent unless it has had at least three weeks at the appropriate dose without indication of response. By the same token, once effective, antidepressants should not be discontinued prematurely. A National Institute of Mental Health collaborative study indicates that they should be continued for 16 to 20 weeks after a patient is completely free of symptoms (3). Patients with recurrent depressions should have their medication continued even longer or perhaps even chronically.

The decision on continuation of treatment depends on the following:

1. How predictable are the episodes?
2. Will the patient be able to seek treatment rapidly if symptoms recur?
3. How much warning does the patient have before getting into serious difficulty?

Patients who become suicidal early in the course of an episode should be treated more aggressively than patients who have several weeks of early morning awakening as a prodrome. Patients who become overwhelmed with hopelessness and are therefore less likely to engage in treatment should also have more extended prophylaxis. It is important that every effort be made to prevent relapse as repeat episodes are associated with a significant chance of developing into chronicity (4).

### BIPOLAR DISORDER, DEPRESSED PHASE

Treatment of the depressed phase of bipolar disorder illustrates the need to distinguish between treatment of an acute episode and prophylaxis. Lithium and carbamazepine are very effective agents for preventing the return of either depression or mania, but both are relatively ineffective in the treatment of a depressive episode. Bipolar patients in the depressed phase should be treated as unipolar depressives, differing only in that antidepressants or ECT pose the risk of inducing a manic episode. Depressed patients who have manic episodes induced by biological treatment are said to have type II bipolar disorder. Patients with past or family history of mania are especially vulnerable. Patients with previous history of antidepressant-induced mania should have lithium or carbamazepine coadministered with the antidepressant. Other patients at risk warrant at least a watchful eye for the development of mania.

### DYSTHYMIA

The data supporting use of antidepressants with these patients are far more equivocal. Dysthymia is by definition a chronic disorder, and this does not augur well for response. Antidepressant therapy should, nonetheless, be tried; a significant percentage of these patients do respond.

### ADJUSTMENT DISORDER WITH DEPRESSED MOOD

Formerly there was a distinction made between "reactive" and "endogenous" depression. This terminology is entering into disuse. The key concept is that the predictors described earlier hold true whether the depression is secondary to a major loss or occurs without clear precipitating events. Many recent widows will have diminished appetite and libido, insomnia, and depressed mood. Acutely, this is a perfectly appropriate part of the grieving process. Such patients should obviously not be medicated. There can come a point, however, when the grieving process has gone on too long and no resolution appears to be forthcoming. This is the time when antidepressants have a role—not to make the grief disappear, but to facilitate the necessary mourning that will allow someone to resume his or her life. The art is in deciding when this point has occurred. There is no exact answer to this question.

### ATYPICAL DEPRESSION

MAOIs may be helpful for the same depressive indications as HCAs. In addition, they have been advocated in a wide variety of "atypical" depressions. These various syndromes all seem to have significant anxiety as a common feature. Reactivity of mood, hypersomnia, hyperphagia, lethargy, and sensitivity to rejection have also been pinpointed as characteristics increasing the likelihood of MAOI response (5). MAOIs are both good antidepressants and anxiolytics if used for a sufficient period at an adequate dose.

### *PANIC DISORDER*

The pharmacological treatment of panic disorder is discussed in Chapter 8. MAOIs, certain atypical benzodiazepines, and all HCAs that have been studied, with the exception of trazodone, have proved effective in preventing panic attacks.

### *OBSESSIVE COMPULSIVE DISORDER*

Clomipramine is peculiarly effective with obsessive compulsive patients. This is discussed in Chapter 8.

### *CHRONIC PAIN SYNDROMES*

Low doses of antidepressants can be used both as adjuncts to analgesics and for a more direct analgesic effect. This is discussed in Chapter 8.

### *EATING DISORDERS*

Patients with bulimia, but not with restrictive anorexia, appear to respond to both HCA and MAOI antidepressants. See Chapter 8.

### *SUBSTANCE ABUSE*

Antidepressants can facilitate withdrawal from cocaine. Data are more conflicted with alcoholics. Both are covered in Chapter 8.

## ■ BASIC PHARMACOLOGY

### *HETEROCYCLICS*

The HCAs include tetra-, tri-, bi-, and unicyclic antidepressants, distinguished by the number of rings in their chemical structure.

There is as much as a tenfold variation in steady-state plasma levels among individuals. This is primarily due to variation in hepatic microenzyme activity, which is largely determined genetically. The drugs are well absorbed after oral administration and are tightly bound to alpha$_1$-glycoproteins and albumin. Since only free, unbound drug permeates the blood–brain barrier and is therefore psychoactive, minor changes in these plasma proteins can have a major impact. The alpha$_1$-glycoproteins are said to be stress related, with an increase being noted with physical illness or other stress. Although there are theoretical reasons to think that the amount of free, or active, drug would decline in the face of stress, there is no clinically meaningful documentation of such an effect. Plasma tricyclic levels reflect the total amount of drug, bound and unbound, and therefore may not always predict clinical efficacy (see Table 2). Patients with atypical binding may well be outliers who respond at "nontherapeutic" blood levels. Nonetheless, plasma levels can be quite helpful in arriving at the appropriate doses for some of these drugs.

The technique for determining a plasma level is relatively simple. Blood should be obtained 12 hours after the last dose in order to reflect trough values. Levels should not be drawn on a patient who is doing well; if, for some reason, this were done, then the clinician should be guided by the patient's course and not the

TABLE 2. **Tricyclic Plasma Levels**

| Advantages | Disadvantages |
|---|---|
| 1. There are good data correlating level and response for three drugs:<br>a. Imipramine—total for imipramine + desipramine > 225 ng/ml<br>b. Desipramine > 125 ng/ml<br>c. Nortriptyline > 50–150 ng/ml<br>2. For unresponsive or unusually toxic patients, levels allow determination of appropriate dosing. | 1. There are conflicting data for all other heterocyclic antidepressants.<br>2. These data are for populations only. Any given patient could be an outlier.<br>3. It is a technically difficult assay. Know your lab. |

numbers. If a patient fails to respond or manifests significant toxicity, then the test can be of great value. For nortriptyline there is convincing evidence of a "therapeutic window." The dose–response curve is curvilinear, so that having too high a level is just as likely to be associated with nonresponse as having too low a level. The remaining two drugs for which there are good data, imipramine and desipramine, have linear responses; a level anywhere above the threshold will be associated with response, although overshooting by too wide a margin will increase the likelihood of toxicity. Most laboratories will quote "therapeutic" levels for a number of other HCAs, but considerable skepticism should be invoked since data on all other compounds are quite conflicted (6).

## *INTERACTIONS*

Certain interactions and predictors of levels are worth attending to. Levels are increased by coadministration of drugs that inhibit the cytochrome P-450 system, such as chlorpromazine, perhaps other antipsychotics, disulfiram, cimetidine, estrogens, and methylphenidate. They are also higher for blacks than whites and are increased by weight loss. They are decreased by oral contraceptives, smoking and barbiturates (7).

## *MECHANISM OF ACTION*

Even if dosed appropriately, there will still be a two- to three-week lag before the antidepressant effect will be evident. The delay in response is, unfortunately, shared by all biological treatments for depression. This leads to suggestions about the mechanism of action of antidepressant treatments.

The old biogenic amine theory held that depression reflected decreased levels of norepinephrine (NE) and serotonin (5-hydroxytryptamine or 5-HT) and that mania reflected an increase in these two neurotransmitters. Antidepressants were seen as effective because they blocked reuptake of these transmitters, leading to increased amounts of both. This thesis suffers from two flaws: 1) Certain atypical, but effective, antidepressants do not block reuptake of NE and 5-HT, and 2) it does not account for the latency of response. Moreover, while most antidepressants do increase NE and 5-HT, they do so acutely, well before any effect is clinically apparent, so some other explanation must be invoked.

No single theory satisfactorily explains all antidepressant therapies. It may, in fact, be that drug *X* operates differently from drug *Y*, but certain generalities probably hold true. The lag between initial administration and response is consistent with the time required to alter receptor sensitivity. Chronic, but not acute, administration of any biological antidepressant therapy will be associated with decreased sensitivity (down-regulation) of the beta-adrenergic receptor. This would seem a sufficient explanation were it not for its lack of specificity: Chlorpromazine and amphetamine have the same effect and are not terribly helpful in the treatment of depression. Long-term, but not acute, treatment seems to be associated with up-regulation of the postsynaptic $alpha_1$ receptor and desensitization of the inhibitory, autoregulatory presynaptic $alpha_2$ receptor. The net result is the release of more NE per impulse and increased impact at the effector receptor. There seems to be a parallel process at the 5-HT receptor as well (8). It may well be that different antidepressants operate by different mechanisms and that this accounts for some patients' responding to one antidepressant but not to another.

At one point, the latter view was widely held, and patients were routinely tried on a serotonergic drug or an adrenergic drug then switched to the other class if the first failed. Various lists order drugs as to serotonergic and adrenergic activity, but reality is less pure. Amitriptyline is usually noted as primarily serotonergic, yet its metabolite, nortriptyline, is considerably more adrenergic and the ratio of the two compounds in vivo will vary considerably. There still may be some rationale for such a switch, but it usually makes more sense to try a more radically different approach, such as lithium augmentation, an MAOI, or ECT.

## *MONOAMINE OXIDASE INHIBITORS*

The MAOIs act through inactivation of the outer mitochondrial enzyme monoamine oxidase. While MAOIs' plasma half-lives are measured in hours, their biologic half-life will last for weeks. This reflects the fact that they will continue to exert an influence until the enzyme has had time to regenerate, which will typically take two weeks, although isolated case reports exist implying that the impact can be a month or more for some. This represents one of the great problems with MAOIs: When they are unsuccessful the clinician's hands are tied for a long time. Patients must be off the drug for at least two weeks before it is safe to try either ECT or a heterocyclic. Work is being conducted in an attempt to find a substance that will block the enzyme, yet reverse readily. There will be considerably greater flexibility and safety once such drugs are available.

There are two types of monoamine oxidase, *MAO-A* and *MAO-B*. Distinctions between the two are relative and not absolute. MAO-A deaminates serotonin, norepinepherine, and epinepherine. MAO-B acts on dopamine. Experimental agents, such as clorgyline, that primarily affect MAO-A are more effective antidepressants than those like pargyline, which preferentially inhibit MAO-B. The usual MAOIs used as antidepressants are nonselective and effect both subtypes. Both MAO-A and MAO-B cleave tyramine and tryptamine. Tyramine is a potent pressor that is normally inactivated by MAO in the gut. If the enzyme is blocked and tyramine is ingested, there is the risk of hypertensive crisis. It is for this reason that patients on these drugs must be on a tyramine-free diet.

At one time, there was considerable enthusiasm about platelet MAO activity, based on the theory that this was an easily accessible reflection of the enzyme's activity in brain. There is some crude correlation with phenelzine's antidepressant activity increasing with 85% or more inhibition of platelet MAO activity. The limitations of this approach may reflect the fact that platelet MAO activity is MAO-B, whereas most of the antidepressant effect reflects inhibition of MAO-A.

One of the advantages of MAOIs is their relative selectivity. They are essentially devoid of effect on the muscarinic receptor and are therefore frequently used with patients who are sensitive to anticholinergic toxicities. The lack of cholinergic impact is also shared with trazodone and fluoxitene, as is an absence of effect on conduction. They are also unlikely to induce arrythmia. The usual dose-limiting factor is orthostasis, probably secondary to an effect on alpha-adrenergic receptors.

## ■ DOSE AND DURATION OF TREATMENT

The most common error is prescribing inadequate amounts of these drugs for an inadequate period. Subtherapeutic doses expose patients to potential toxicity without the opportunity for benefit; treating for less than three to four weeks often leads to prematurely abandoning a potentially helpful agent.

For HCAs there is as much as a tenfold difference in dose and plasma level among individual patients. Table 3 lists normative doses, but it must be realized that many patients fall outside of these ranges. It is for this reason that drugs that have good data correlating plasma level and response are to be preferred. Particular note should also be taken of the compounds with atypical doses: Nortriptyline and protriptyline are more potent than most, amoxapine and trazodone less. Normally, all HCAs can be given at bedtime. Trazodone may need to be split during the day because of its very short plasma half-life. Large doses at bedtime can occasionally be accompanied by nightmares; if this is the case, then the dose should be split. Single nighttime doses can also be a problem for the patient who gets up suddenly during the night to go to the bathroom; here orthostasis can pose a difficulty. All HCAs with the exception of protriptyline (which should be given in the morning) are typically sedating. Prescription at night is an example of attempting to benefit from toxicity.

A patient should be started on an HCA gradually. If a full treatment dose is begun right away both the $alpha_2$ and anticholinergic toxicities may be more than the patient can tolerate. It usually makes sense to start the patient with 50 mg of imipramine or equivalent and increase by a similar quantity every three to four days. The dose can then be held at 150 or 200 mg, depending on the patient's size and tolerance for another one to two weeks in order to monitor for response.

A reasonable guideline for dosing phenelzine (brand name: Nardil) is to aim for 1 mg per kg of body weight. The usual range is 45 to 90 mg q.d. Tranylcypromine (brand name: Parnate) may be thought of as twice as potent. Both drugs, but particularly tranylcypromine, are usually mildly activating. For this reason they should be taken in the morning, typically in a split dose. The dose should be gradually increased in much the same fashion as HCAs.

TABLE 3. **Heterocyclic Antidepressants**

| Class/Generic Name | Brand Name | Half-Life (Hours) | Usual Dosage (mg) | Therapeutic Plasma Level ng/ml | Comments |
|---|---|---|---|---|---|
| Tertiary tricyclics | | | | | |
| Amitriptyline[a] | Elavil, Endep, others | 16 | 150–300 | | |
| Doxepin[a] | Adapin, Sinequan | 17 | 150–300 | | Quite sedating |
| Imipramine[a] | Tofranil, SK-Pramine, Janimine, others | 22 | 150–300 | Total imipramine + desipramine > 225 | |
| Trimipramine | Surmontil | 9 | 150–300 | Unknown | Very sedating, but little anticholinergic effect |
| Secondary tricyclics | | | | | |
| Desipramine | Norpramine | 21 | 150–300 | > 125 | First-pass metabolite of imipramine |
| Nortriptyline | Aventyl, Pamelor | 27 | 75–150 | 50–150 | First-pass metabolite of amitriptyline |
| Protriptyline | Vivactil | 78 | 10–40 | Unknown | The most activating heterocyclic |

| | | | | | |
|---|---|---|---|---|---|
| Dibenzoxazepine | | | | | |
| Amoxapine | Asendin | 30 | 100–400 | Unknown | Blocks dopamine receptors and has risk of tardive dyskinesia, extrapyramidal symptoms, and galactorrhea |
| Tetracyclic | | | | | |
| Maprotiline | Ludiomil | 47 | 150–300 | Unknown | Increased incidence of seizures; 3% develop a skin rash |
| Triazolopyridine | | | | | |
| Trazodone[a] | Desyrel | 5 | 100–600 | Unknown | Sedating; does not extend conduction deficits; does increase ventricular ectopy and cause priapism; safe overdoses |
| Bicyclic | | | | | |
| Fluoxetine | Prozac | 72 | 40–80 | Unknown | Pure serotonergic drug; does not interact with alcohol; weight *loss* noted; little orthostasis; somewhat activating |

[a] Available generically.

For both MAOIs and HCAs there must be a minimum of three to four weeks at adequate dose before they should be considered a failure. If after such a period there are early signs of response, then they should be continued, since it often takes six weeks for the maximal response to be evident.

The risk of relapse is greatest in the first several months after discontinuation of antidepressants. Because of this it is probably prudent to continue a patient recovering from a first episode of depression for 16 to 20 weeks after he or she is symptom free (3). For bipolar patients, lithium has been shown to have superior efficacy over HCAs. For unipolar patients, the results are comparable. In the presence of a family history of bipolar disorder, lithium is preferred; absent such a history, the physician would be wise to opt for whichever agent would lead to enhanced compliance. Recurrent patients should have medication maintained for several times their average cycle length before it is withdrawn (9).

## ■ SIDE EFFECTS

Both HCAs and MAOIs share certain toxicities, some peculiar to a given class and some limited to certain agents within each group. All antidepressants share a relatively low therapeutic index. All of them can be used to commit *suicide*. Since patients with depression are at high risk, some physicians avoid prescription of the very agents that could be of help to them. Such a blanket prohibition is not warranted, but patients should be routinely asked about suicide ideation. Except in unusual situations, prescriptions should not be written for more than a one-week supply with patients who have any thoughts of suicide. Admittedly, patients can cache away several weeks' worth, but writing a limited supply prevents impulsive acting-out and forces the physician to reevaluate the patient frequently. Particular caution should be exercised as patients are starting to emerge from an episode. This is when suicide potential often maximizes, probably reflecting the asynchrony of response to antidepressants; energy often responds before suicide ideation, leaving patients able to act.

There is renewed debate about whether biologic treatment of depression carries the risk of inducing *mania*. Clearly, some patients who are receiving antidepressant therapy cycle into manic episodes. What is less clear is whether this happens more often than would occur without any intervention. The data on this are conflicting, but some individuals do cycle as a result of treatment and should have lithium or carbamazepine prophylaxis. Patients are at particular risk by virtue of past history of mania, family history of mania, or prior episodes of drug-induced cycling.

## *HETEROCYCLIC ANTIDEPRESSANT SIDE EFFECTS*

Understanding which receptors are affected will go a long way toward predicting toxicities associated with particular agents. Table 4 lists these data. The information in Table 4 should be correlated with that in Table 5, which notes the signs and

TABLE 4. **Heterocyclic Antidepressants and Receptors**

| Generic Name | Anti-cholinergic Affinity | $Alpha_1$ Affinity | Histamine $H_1$ Affinity |
|---|---|---|---|
| Amitriptyline | 4 | 3 | 3 |
| Amoxapine | 1 | 2 | 1 |
| Clomipramine[a,b] | 2 | — | 0 |
| Desipramine | 1 | 1 | 0 |
| Doxepin | 2 | 3 | 4 |
| Fluoxetine[b,c] | 0 | 1/0 | 0 |
| Imipramine | 2 | 1 | 1 |
| Maprotiline[d] | 1 | 1 | 2 |
| Mianserin[a,d] | 0/1 | — | — |
| Nortriptyline | 1 | 1 | 1 |
| Protriptyline | 3 | 1 | 0 |
| Trazodone[b] | 0 | 2 | 0 |
| Trimipramine | 2 | 3 | 4 |

*Note.* 0 = no effect; 4 = maximal effect. Adapted from Sulser F: Pharmacology: current antidepressants. Psychiatric Annals 1980; 10:526-534; Feigner JP: Clinical efficacy of the newer antidepressants. J. Clin Psychopharmacol 1982; 1:23S-26S; Richardson JM, Richelson E: Antidepressants: a clinical update for medical practitioners. Mayo Clin Proc 1984; 59:330-337; and Richelson E: Are receptor studies useful for clinical practice? J Clin Psychiatry 1983; 44:4-9

[a] Not yet approved by the Food and Drug Administration.
[b] Triazolopyridine.
[c] Bicyclic.
[d] Tetracyclic.

TABLE 5. **Antidepressant Side Effects According to Receptor Sites**

| |
|---|
| Anticholinergic |
| Sedation, drowsiness |
| Delirium |
| Visual blurring |
| Exacerbation of narrow-angle glaucoma |
| Xerostomia (dry mouth)—can lead to caries and stomatitis |
| Constipation |
| Urinary retention and hesitancy |
| Sexual dysfunction |
| Cognitive dysfunction |
| Increased heart rate |
| Antihistamine $H_1$ |
| Sedation |
| Weight gain |
| Alpha blockade |
| Postural hypotension |
| Reflex tachycardia |
| Miscellaneous or unknown mechanism |
| Tremor |
| Edema |

symptoms associated with involvement of particular sets of receptors. It then becomes easy to predict that amitriptyline is quite sedating on the basis of its strong antihistaminic effect.

## ANTICHOLINERGIC EFFECTS

Anticholinergic effects are generally most evident during the first months of use. Patients will often accommodate after this. These tend to be greatest with the tertiary tricyclics (amitriptyline, imipramine, trimipramine, doxepin) and less for their demethylated metabolites. If patients are unable to tolerate them, then a switch to the less anticholinergic metabolite may make sense.

Xerostomia, or *dry mouth*, can lead to stomatitis or caries. Increased fluid intake and sugarless candies or gum are often sufficient treatment. If they are not, then bethanechol 10–30 mg q.d.–b.i.d. may be added (10).

*Blurring for near vision* secondary to mydriasis and

cycloplegia also occurs. Patients should not rush to have their prescriptions changed unless they are to stay on a stable dose for a prolonged period. Bethanechol can again be helpful, or pilocarpine 1% opthalmic solution one drop q.i.d. can be administered. Patients with shallow anterior chambers are at risk for *acute narrow-angle glaucoma* if exposed to drugs that limit accommodation. Patients should be screened for this defect with the penlight test. A penlight is shined across the eye; if the nasal side of the iris fails to illuminate, then the patient is at some potential risk and should have his or her intraocular pressure checked (11).

*Constipation* is best managed with bran, a bulk laxative, or a stool softener.

Elderly patients with enlarged prostates are at particular risk for the development of *urinary retention.* If severe, there may be the need for referral to a urologist. If there is merely some urinary hesitation, then bethanechol can be helpful.

A wide variety of *sexual difficulties* have been cited. Libido has been reported as both decreased and increased. The latter is more usually the case, since diminished sexual interest can be one of the targets for antidepressants. Priapism has been reported with trazodone. The drug should be discontinued and urologic intervention promptly requested if an erection does not cease. Erectile dysfunction and ejaculatory disturbance will generally respond to switching to a less anticholinergic antidepressant.

The most subtle, difficult-to-diagnose toxicities are *mental status changes.* Frank delirium usually occurs when these medications are combined with other anticholinergic agents. Typically, some of the other stigmata of anticholinergic excess are evident (tachycardia, flushed facies, thirst, dry mucous membranes, enlarged pupils), but occasionally nothing is seen save mental changes. While most patients experience improvement in memory as the depression lifts, some elderly, cognitively compromised patients may have memory difficulties exacerbated with the addition of these agents. If a patient's memory worsens, then cautious withdrawal of the antidepressant should be contemplated.

## ANTIHISTAMINIC EFFECTS

*Sedation* is an example of a side effect that may be turned to the patient's advantage. Drugs that are potent antihistamines should be given at bedtime in order to assist with sleep.

*Weight gain* can be a problem for patients on both MAOIs and tricyclics. The mechanism is unknown, although speculation centers on an antihistaminic effect. It does not appear to simply reflect improvement of the anorexia associated with depression, because nondepressed panic-disordered patients are vulnerable to this as well. Unfortunately, there have not been good trials comparing various antidepressants, but the common practice is to switch to a less antihistaminic antidepressant if weight gain is a major problem. Fluoxitene appears to be associated with weight loss.

Although not a toxicity, there is one further antihistaminic effect that should be noted. Both controlled and open trials support the in vitro data that trimipramine and doxepin are potent *$H_2$ antagonists*. They have compared favorably with ranitidine and cimetidine. Either of these agents can probably be discontinued in favor of these antidepressants (12).

## ALPHA EFFECTS

Orthostatic, or postural, hypotension often impinges on antidepressant treatment, particularly in elderly, cardiovascularly compromised patients. Generally, there is more risk with tertiary tricyclics. Curiously, this liability appears dose related with MAOIs but not with HCAs.

Baseline orthostatic readings should always be obtained prior to the prescription of antidepressants. Readings should be repeated over 5 to 10 minutes after the patient stands. Without baseline readings, the physician is often left with the assumption that the medication is causing the postural change when other factors could be responsible. Table 6 lists some of the other common etiologies.

Patients at risk should have tertiary tricyclics prescribed. Nortriptyline and desipramine are particularly benign. Symptomatic treatment may still be necessary. Restoration of fluid volume, raising the head of the bed, waist-high elastic support stockings, or liberalized salt intake may be enough (13). All patients should be instructed to get up slowly from either lying or sitting. They should learn to dangle their legs over the side of the bed for several minutes before arising.

It should be remembered that it is symptoms, not numbers, that matter. Treatment should be contemplated if patients com-

TABLE 6. **Common Causes of Orthostasis**

| |
|---|
| Diabetes mellitus |
| Parkinson's disease |
| Addison's disease |
| Shy-Drager syndrome |
| Amyloidosis |
| Prolonged bedrest |
| Pregnancy |
| Varicose veins |
| Antihypertensive medication |
| Alpha-adrenergic antagonists |
| Arrhythmia |
| Volume depletion: dehydration, hemorrhage, etc. |

plain of lightheadedness or syncope. Many patients will be entirely asymptomatic even in the face of a 30-point drop in systolic blood pressure. Symptomatic patients who fail to respond to conservative measures may benefit from the addition of 9-alpha-fludrocortisone (Florinef), a mineralocorticoid that is begun at 0.1 mg q.d.–b.i.d. and titrated up every five to seven days to doses as high as 1.0 mg q.d. The chief risks are hypokalemia, congestive heart failure, and hypertension. All should be regularly monitored (14).

## MISCELLANEOUS EFFECTS

A fine, nonparkinsonian *tremor* has been noted, especially with the more adrenergic HCAs. Discontinuation of caffeine and tobacco is frequently helpful. If symptoms persist, it may be justified to treat with a peripherally acting beta-blocker.

*Edema* can occur. The mechanism is unknown, but has been noted in the absence of other signs of heart failure. Symptomatic treatment with low doses of a thiazide can be helpful.

*Myoclonus*, especially as patients are falling asleep, can occur with both HCAs and MAOIs (15). This may reflect serotonergic activity and is frequently dose related. It is annoying but not dangerous. Treatment alternatives include dose reduction, change to a less serotonergic drug, or symptomatic treatment with clonazepam 0.5–1.5 mg at bedtime.

## *MONOAMINE OXIDASE INHIBITOR SIDE EFFECTS*

MAOIs have minimal anticholinergic or antihistaminic effect. They are potent alpha-blockers and, in addition, have problems that are direct results of inhibition of the enzyme. The predictable problems with orthostasis are the usual dose-limiting factors. Their minimal impact on muscarinic receptors, their lack of effect on cardiac conduction, and the increase in MAO activity that is seen with advanced age are making them more and more attractive to geropsychiatrists.

### MONOAMINE OXIDASE INHIBITION

Monoamine oxidase is normally present in the gut as well as brain. One of its functions is to inactivate various pressors, notably tyramine which is widely distributed in various foodstuffs. If these pressor agents are not inactivated, a dramatic increase in blood pressure can result. It is for this reason that patients must follow a special low-tyramine diet and must also be aware of the many potential interactions with prescribed and over-the-counter medications.

Many of the low-tyramine diets that have been published are overly restrictive, largely reflecting medical folklore rather than data. Patients often experiment, find that they can get away with it, and then go further, resulting in serious difficulty. The dietary suggestions listed in Table 7 attempt to order foods into low, moderate, and high tyramine content. Patients should be instructed to completely avoid any foods listed as moderate or higher. Other foods may be enjoyed in moderation.

Drug interactions need to be considered as well (see Table 8). They are discussed in the section on interactions. Many over-the-counter medications contain sympathomimetics and should be avoided. Patients should be instructed to not take any new medication until they have checked with their physician.

It is imperative that patients be properly educated as to the risks of MAOIs. They are quite safe if used appropriately, but patients must be capable of understanding and following the diet or must be in a structured setting that will ensure compliance.

TABLE 7. **Tyramine in Food and Beverages**

| Food or Beverage | Estimated Levels[a] |
|---|---|
| Cheese | |
| American, processed | Low |
| Blue | Moderate to high |
| Boursault | Very high |
| Brick, natural | Moderate to high |
| Brie | Moderate to high |
| Camembert | Very high |
| Cheddar | Very high |
| Cottage cheese | Little or none |
| Cream cheese | Little or none |
| Emmenthaler | Very high |
| Gruyere | Moderate to high |
| Mozzarella | Moderate to high |
| Parmesan | Moderate to high |
| Romano | Moderate to high |
| Roquefort | Moderate to high |
| Stilton | Very high |
| Meat and fish | |
| Beef liver, unrefrigerated, fermented | Moderate |
| Caviar | High |
| Chicken liver, unrefrigerated, fermented | Moderate |
| Fish, unrefrigerated, fermented | Moderate |
| Fish, dried | Moderate |
| Herring, dried salted | Moderate to high |
| Herring, pickled, if spoiled | Highest levels found |
| Sausages, fermented | Very high |
| Bologna | |
| Pepperoni | |
| Salami | |
| Summer sausage | |
| Other unrefrigerated, fermented meats | Moderate |
| Beverages | |
| Beer and Ale[b] | Low (up to 10 $\mu$g/ml) |
| Chartreuse[c] | Unknown |
| Drambuie[c] | Unknown |
| Sherry[c] | Low |
| Wine, red[d] | Low |
| Wine, white[e] | Little or none |
| Nonalcoholic beer, lager | 0.8 $\mu$g/ml |

*(cont.)*

TABLE 7. **Tyramine in Food and Beverages** *(continued)*

| Food or Beverage | Estimated Levels[a] |
|---|---|
| Vegetables | |
| Avocado, particularly if overripe | Low to moderate |
| Fava beans, particularly if overripe | Contain dopamine |
| New Zealand prickly spinach (large amounts)[c] | Unknown |
| Fruits | |
| Bananas | Low |
| Figs, canned, particularly if overripe | Low to moderate |
| Others | |
| Caffeine, very large amounts | A weak pressor agent |
| Chocolate, very large amounts | Contains phenylethylamine, a weak pressor agent |
| Yeast extracts such as Marmite[f] | Very high |

[a] The tyramine content of most foods is not entirely predictable. These estimates are taken from isolated reports, some based on small samples. The amount of tyramine in food and beverages could vary with different conditions, different samples, and different manufacturers.

[b] Fermentation of beer does not ordinarily involve processes that produce tyramine. Some imported beers have caused reactions in patients taking inhibitors.

[c] Some patients have had reactions.

[d] Fermentation of wine does not ordinarily produce tyramine. However, contamination with other than the usual fermenting organisms and production of appreciable amounts of tyramine has occurred in Chianti and could occur in any red wine.

[e] White wine is free of tyramine because it is made without the grape pulp and seeds, which may be the source of amino acids in red wine.

[f] However, baked goods do not contain appreciable amounts of tyramine.

From *The Medical Letter Handbook of Adverse Drug Interactions, 1985*. New Rochelle, NY, The Medical Letter, 1985. Reprinted with the permission of the publisher.

Patients should examine the dietary restrictions before electing to receive these drugs.

*Hypertensive crises* are, fortunately, quite rare. Patients should know the symptoms associated with the reaction, including a throbbing, intense headache; flushing; nausea and vomiting; photophobia; and palpitations. If these symptoms occur patients should promptly seek medical attention. Such patients can be treated with phentolamine 5.0 mg IV. Patients who do not have easy access to medical care would do well to carry a 50 mg tablet of chlorpromazine with them. Its alpha-blocking properties make this an effective stopgap measure.

TABLE 8. **Monoamine Oxidase Inhibitor Drug Interactions, Mechanism, and Alternatives**

| Drug | Result and Mechanism | Alternatives |
|---|---|---|
| Meperidine | Encephalopathy, unknown mechanism | Aspirin, acetaminophen, nonsteroidal anti-inflammatory agents, codeine, oxycodone |
| Dextromethorphan | Unknown mechanism; single case report of hyperpyrexia and death; potentially hypertensive crisis | Guaifenesin elixir (Robitussin), terpin hydrate with codeine |
| Buspirone | Increased norepinephrine | Benzodiazepines |
| Heterocyclic antidepressants (HCAs) | Fever, seizures, mechanism unknown | Two-week washout in going from an MAOI to an HCA; one week in going the other way |
| Sympathomimetics[a] | Hypertensive crisis | |
| | Cold, rhinitis | Antihistamines (brompheniramine, chlorpheniramine) |
| | Obesity | Exercise, diet |
| | Anesthesia | For local, use non-epinephrine-containing lidocaine or procaine; for major surgery, washout two weeks in advance; in an emergency, correct hypotension with fluids; avoid succinylcholine |
| Succinylcholine | Prolonged muscle relaxation | See above |
| Electroconvulsive therapy | Potential hypertension due to increased catecholamines | Washout two weeks before |
| Methyldopa | Hypotension | Diuretics |
| Clonidine | | Vasodilators |
| High-dose beta-blockers | | Angiotensin conventing enzyme inhibitors |
| Guanethidine | | |
| Reserpine | | |

[a] Amphetamine, l-dopa, ephedrine, epinephrine, isoproterenol, metaraminol, methylphenidate, norepinephrine, phenylephrine, phenylpropanolamine, pseudoephedrine, and others.

**MISCELLANEOUS MONOAMINE OXIDASE INHIBITOR TOXICITIES**

Women may note dose-related *anorgasmia.*

Many patients find these drugs, particularly tranylcypromine, to be activating and associated with *sleep interruption.* This can be avoided by giving the medicine in a split dose early in the day.

*Paresthesias* have been reported. They often respond to pyridoxine.

## *CARDIOVASCULAR EFFECTS*

The effects on blood pressure have already been reviewed. There is also an increase in *heart rate*, probably related to the anticholinergic effect. Since MAOIs have less anticholinergic effect, there is less associated tachycardia. Increased heart rate can be problematic for patients with unstable angina or marginally compensated congestive heart failure (16).

All HCAs with the exception of trazodone will *prolong cardiac conduction* much like quinidine, procainamide, or disopyramide. Trials have favorably compared imipramine with these type I antiarrhythmics. Patients receiving HCAs can often have their quinidine or procainamide discontinued or have the dose substantially lowered. They do carry the risk of extending any conduction abnormality. Patients with low-grade conduction abnormalities such as a first-degree atrioventricular block, a Mobitz type I second-degree atrioventricular block, a right bundle branch block, or a left anterior hemiblock should have only very cautious use of an HCA, with all dose increases accompanied by serial electrocardiograms. With these patients, trazodone, an MAOI, or ECT may make more sense. Patients with higher block (bifasicular or Mobitz type II second-degree atrioventricular blocks) should not have HCAs with the exception of trazodone or fluoxitene under any circumstances. Trazodone has been associated with an increase in ventricular ectopy. Doxepin has been advocated by some as having less cardiovascular toxicity, but this appears to be an artifact of trials with low doses. MAOIs are remarkably well tolerated, with the exception of the associated postural hypotension. There are no data supporting any important effect of MAOIs on conduction or rhythm.

## *MANAGEMENT OF OVERDOSE*

### HETEROCYCLICS

Virtually any arrythmia can be seen. Stuporous patients or patients with respiratory insufficiency, seizures, arrythmia, or a QRS interval of greater than 100 ms should have electrocardiogram telemetry. The prolonged QRS interval correlates with very high, potentially lethal plasma levels. While the anticholinergic effect can decrease gastric motility and slow absorption, and while lipophilicity also contributes to a delayed effect, no patients have been reported to get into trouble once they have regained alertness and their electrocardiograms have normalized. The delay in absorption necessitates gastric lavage, cathartics, and charcoal. Seizures are treated symptomatically with intravenous benzodiazepines. Intubation may be necessary. Arrhythmia should be treated with sodium bicarbonate and beta-blockers. Lidocaine may be used as required. Type I antiarrhythmics should be avoided because they will increase the arrhythmogenic effects of the HCA. Pacemakers and Swan-Ganz catheters may be required. Most deaths are cardiac and occur within the first 24 hours. They are usually associated with doses in excess of 1250 mg of imipramine or equivalent.

### MONOAMINE OXIDASE INHIBITORS

Toxicity is usually manifested by central nervous system hyperactivity with agitation, hyperreflexia, and rigidity. Both hyper- and hypotension have been reported. Death, coma, and arrhythmia are all rare.

# ■ WITHDRAWAL OF ANTIDEPRESSANTS

## *HETEROCYCLICS*

Abrupt discontinuation of an antidepressant can be associated either with the development of a withdrawal syndrome or with reemergence of the depression. Because of this the medications should be gradually tapered in an attempt to establish if there is a lower, effective dose. Withdrawal effects can include anxiety, restlessness, diarrhea, piloerection, and, rarely, delirium and mania (17).

### *MONOAMINE OXIDASE INHIBITORS*

Evidence for a withdrawal syndrome is lacking, although the comments above about reemergent depression hold true here as well. It must be remembered that it will take two weeks for MAO to regenerate. Patients must maintain their diets and be wary of interactions for this period.

## ■ INTERACTIONS

### *MONOAMINE OXIDASE INHIBITOR AND HETEROCYCLIC USE*

For populations of patients, there are no data indicating that coprescription is any better than either drug alone. It is clear, however, that individual patients refractory to both drugs can respond to the combination. If precautions are not taken this can be a very dangerous combination resulting in hyperpyrexia, convulsions, tremor, increased tone, and coma. If guidelines are followed the combination can be managed safely (18). *HCAs should never be added to an MAOI without an intervening two-week washout.* Ideally, there should be a medication-free period followed by concurrent initiation of the antidepressants. The favored HCAs are amitriptyline, doxepin, and trimipramine. Imipramine and desipramine should not be used. Phenelzine is the choice over tranylcypromine. Doses should be gradually increased. The final doses are dependent on the outcome, but full antidepressant regimens of both are frequently required. This approach is best reserved for the patient who fails to respond to more conventional regimens.

### *HETEROCYCLICS*

HCAs are metabolized via the cytochrome P-450 system. Other drugs that are metabolized in this way (phenothiazines, alcohol, cimetidine, disulfiram, oral contraceptives) will result in increased levels of both if coadministered. Smoking and barbiturates induce the same system and result in lower levels. This is not problematic if the doses of all drugs remain constant. It simply means that less of the drugs will be required once past the loading stage.

HCAs act by blocking reuptake into the presynaptic neuron. This means that antihypertensives such as guanethidine will be ineffective. Sympathomimetics will, on the other hand, have a greatly augmented effect to the point where hypertensive crisis may eventuate. This is because their effect is not terminated by reuptake as is usually the case.

Additive effects are predictable with other agents that are anticholinergic or alpha-blockers.

### *MONOAMINE OXIDASE INHIBITORS*

See Table 7 for the interactions with MAOIs.

## ■ AN APPROACH TO THE DEPRESSED PATIENT

A wide variety of treatments are available for depressed patients. Some are more effective than others for particular subpopulations of depressed patients. Moreover, every clinician cannot be equally facile with all of the available treatment options; instead it makes sense to become well acquainted with several of the available alternatives. With this background it becomes clear that there cannot be a broad consensus supporting any particular treatment approach. Each clinician should, however, develop a sequence of treatment options that he or she is comfortable with. The therapies should follow each other logically. The long-range plan should be thought out so that the clinician anticipates what steps would follow if a particular therapeutic approach fails.

What follows is but one series of options. There are considerable grounds for disagreement; many would prefer to try several HCAs before moving on to an MAOI or ECT. This is a perfectly defensible point of view. Rather than suggesting that this is the only appropriate treatment course, the aim here is to suggest that a series of logical options should be entertained from the beginning.

Before beginning, several assumptions about the patient need to be clarified. First, there is an assumption that the correct diagnosis is depression. A structured interview is helpful. At minimum *DSM-III-R* should be used. Diagnosis of melancholia by these criteria is encouraging as a predictor of response. Use of the Hamilton Depression Rating Scale is also helpful (19).

In addition to establishing the diagnosis, a thorough physical and laboratory examination must be done to rule out organic etiologies for the depression and to ensure that the patient can tolerate medication safely.

A careful history should be taken with an eye toward understanding the patient's previous response to medication. Always begin with whichever medication previously worked. If there is no previous antidepressant use, then inquiries should be made about other family members' responses. In the absence of other data, it is prudent to begin with whatever has been helpful for relatives with similar illnesses.

## *SELECTION OF AN INITIAL TREATMENT*

Ordinarily treatment should begin with an HCA. Exceptions would include

1. Past history of response to ECT or an MAOI
2. An atypical depression with hyperphagia, hypersomnolence, anxiety, and emotional hyperactivity
3. Cardiac conduction defects that would suggest fluoxitene, trazodone, an MAOI, or ECT.

If there is no contraindication, use nortriptyline, imipramine, or desipramine, since plasma levels are best developed with these drugs.

Treatment would ordinarily begin with 50 mg of imipramine or desipramine or 25 mg of nortriptyline given at bedtime. If tolerated well, dosage should be increased by a like amount every three days until the patient is taking 200 mg of imipramine or desipramine or 100 mg of nortriptyline at bedtime. If after three weeks there is an insufficient response, then a plasma level should be checked with a reliable laboratory and the dose appropriately titrated. If the patient responds positively, then the medicine should be maintained for 16 to 20 weeks after maximal relief is obtained.

## LITHIUM AUGMENTATION

The nonresponder might benefit from the addition of lithium. The addition of lithium to both HCAs and MAOIs has been helpful to many treatment-refractory patients. Initial investigation was spurred by the fact that lithium serves to increase levels of serotonin. Its role in augmentation seems independent of its function as a thymoleptic since the response is often evident within a week and low doses, along the lines of 300 mg t.i.d., generally prove helpful. Similar results have been obtained with both HCAs and MAOIs (20, 21).

There is considerable reliance on lithium augmentation in this approach. This is because of both its efficacy and the rapidity of response. No more than a week is lost by such an intervention. Although recent data indicate that the full response may well take three weeks, some measure of improvement is usually apparent more rapidly (22). A positive response should lead to maintenance for the same period described previously.

## SECOND-LEVEL TREATMENTS

If a patient fails to respond to these initial treatments, several options could be considered. An MAOI, another HCA, or ECT could all be considered. An MAOI has a reasonably high likelihood of benefit, but significantly limits the available options if it fails. A good trial of an MAOI takes over a month, then a two-week washout has to follow before other treatments can be considered. One HCA may work after another fails, but the likelihood of response is somewhat less than for the other options.

If an MAOI is chosen and the patient fails to respond to three weeks of 1 mg per kg body weight of phenelzine or 0.5 mg per kg of tranylcypromine, then lithium augmentation should be used, as previously described. If this fails, then a two-week washout should be followed by ECT. Patients responding to an MAOI should be maintained for 16 to 20 weeks after maximal improvement.

The small percentage of ECT nonresponders should probably provoke diagnostic reexamination. If such a search confirms the diagnosis of major depression, then a trial of an MAOI should be considered, if not previously attempted. Chapter 5 discusses ECT in detail.

## *THE TREATMENT-REFRACTORY PATIENT*

A depressed patient who fails to respond to the above regimens might be considered truly treatment refractory. A series of alternatives for these patients follows. Each is of relatively low yield for populations of patients, but individuals do respond so that a continued search may well be justified.

### LITHIUM OR CARBAMAZEPINE ALONE

Lithium and carbamazepine both are rather indifferent antidepressants, although they have great value in preventing the return of unipolar depression. In spite of the lack of statistical efficacy in treating populations of depressed patients, they do have a clear value for individuals. They should, however, be consigned to the bottom of the list with other relatively low-yield procedures (23).

### $T_3$ AUGMENTATION

Addition of 25–50 $\mu$g of triiodothyronine to HCAs with treatment-refractory, apparently euthyroid patients has been helpful to some. Curiously, it appears that women are more likely than men to respond to this regimen. There seems to be more of an effect on rate of response, than amount of response (24). Like lithium alone, this is a relatively low-yield procedure.

### TRYPTOPHAN AUGMENTATION

Addition of l-tryptophan, a precursor of serotonin, to MAOIs (but not to HCAs) has been helpful (25). 5-Hydroxytryptophan, another serotonergic precursor, especially if combined with carbidopa, shows promise but is as yet unproven as an antidepressant therapy (26).

### STIMULANTS

In spite of widespread use for depression after their development in the 1930s, there has been remarkably little systematic research on stimulants (27). They have been advocated, especially in medically ill patients intolerant of more conventional antidepressant treatment (28). They are generally well tolerated and are particularly helpful for psychomotorically retarded, apathetic, withdrawn patients. It is less clear whether the effect lasts beyond several weeks, since the few trials in the literature report only on short-term use. The risks include precipitation of a paranoid psychosis, tolerance, insomnia, and anorexia, as well as rebound depression and fatigue with discontinuation of the drug. Trials may nonetheless be warranted in depressed patients unresponsive to more orthodox therapies. The response is usually rapid, so benefit should be apparent within two weeks. The most commonly used agents are dextroamphetamine sulfate 10 to 30 mg q.d. and methylphenidate 10 to 40 mg q.d. Doses should be split and given in the morning to avoid the insomnia associated with their use. The potential for habituation and the lack of controlled support for their use in depression leave them reserved for the treatment-refractory or medically compromised patient intolerant of HCAs or MAOIs.

## ■ REFERENCES


1. DiMascio A, Weissman MM, Prosoff BA, et al: Differential symptom reduction by drugs and psychotherapy in acute depression. Arch Gen Psychiatry 1979; 36:1450-1456
2. American Psychiatric Association: Diagnostic and Statistical Manual of Mental Disorders, Third Edition, Revised. Washington, DC, American Psychiatric Association, 1987
3. Prien RF, Kupfer DJ: Continuation drug therapy for major depressive episodes: how long should it be maintained? Am J Psychiatry 1986; 143:18-23
4. Keller MB, Lavori PW, Rice J, et al: The persistent risk of chronicity in recurrent episodes of nonbipolar major depressive disorder: a prospective follow-up. Am J Psychiatry 1986; 143:224-228
5. Quitkin FM, Harrison W, Liebowitz M, et al: Defining the boundaries of atypical depression. J Clin Psychiatry 1984; 45(suppl):19-21
6. American Psychiatric Association Task Force on the Use of Laboratory Tests in Psychiatry: Tricyclic antidepressants—blood level measurements and clinical outcome: an APA task force report. Am J Psychiatry 1985; 142:155-62
7. Rizack MA, Hillman CDM (eds): The Medical Letter Handbook of Adverse Drug Interactions. New Rochelle, NY, The Medical Letter, 1985
8. Charney DS, Menkes DB, Heninger GB: Receptor sensitivity and the mechanism of action of antidepressant treatment. Arch Gen Psychiatry 1981; 38:1160-1180
9. Consensus Development Panel: Mood disorders: pharmacologic prevention of recurrences. Am J Psychiatry 1985; 142:469-476

10. Pollack MH, Rosenbaum JF: Management of antidepressant-induced side effects: a practical guide for the clinician. J Clin Psychiatry 1987; 48:3-8
11. Lieberman E, Stoudemire A: Use of tricyclic antidepressants in patients with glaucoma. Psychosomatics 1987; 28:145-148
12. Haggerty JJ, Brossman DA: Psychotropic drugs: use in peptic ulcer patients. Psychosomatics 1985; 26:277-284
13. Ornot J, Golberg MR, Hollister AS, et al: Management of chronic orthostatic hypotension. Am J Med 1986; 80:454-464
14. Schatz IJ: Current management concepts in orthostatic hypotension. Arch Intern Med 1980; 1152-1154
15. Garvey M, Tollefson G: Occurrence of myoclonus in patients treated with cyclic antidepressants. Arch Gen Psychiatry 1987; 44:269-272
16. Goldstein MG, Guttmacher LB: Treatment of the cardiac impaired depressed patient: part one. Psychiatric Medicine (in press)
17. Dilsalver SC, Greden JF: Antidepressant withdrawal phenomena. Biol Psychiatry 1984; 19:237-256
18. White K, Simpson G: Combined MAOI–tricyclic antidepressant treatment: a reevaluation. J Clin Psychopharmacol, 1981; 1:264-282
19. Hamilton M: Development of a rating scale for primary depressive illness. Br J Soc Clin Psychol 1967; 6:278-296
20. DeMontigny C, Cournoyer G, Morrissette R, et al: Lithium carbonate addition in tricyclic antidepressant-resistant unipolar depression. Arch Gen Psychiatry 1983; 40:1327-1334
21. Price LH, Charney DS, Heninger GR: Efficacy of lithium–tranylcypromine treatment in refractory depression. Am J Psychiatry 1985; 142:619-623
22. Price LH, Charney DS, Heninger GR: Variability of response to lithium augmentation in refractory depression. Am J Psychiatry 1986; 143:1387-1392
23. Post RM, Uhde TW, Roy-Byrne PP, et al: Antidepressant effects of carbamazepine. Am J Psychiatry 1986; 143:29-34
24. Klein DF, Gittelman R, Quitkin F, et al: Diagnosis and Drug Treatment of Psychiatric Disorders: Adults and Children (second edition). Baltimore, Williams & Wilkins, 1980
25. Van Praag HM: Management of depression with serotonin precursors. Biol Psychiatry 1981; 16:291-310
26. Byerly WF, Judd LL, Reimherr FW, et al: 5-hydroxytryptophan: a review of its antidepressant efficacy and adverse effects. J Clin Psychopharmacol 1987; 7:127-137
27. Chiarello RJ, Cole JO: The use of psychostimulants in general psychiatry. Arch Gen Psychiatry 1987; 44:286-295
28. Kaufmann MW, Murray GB, Cassem NH: Use of psychostimulants in medically ill depressed patients. Psychosomatics 1982; 23:817-819

# AGENTS FOR BIPOLAR DISORDER



## ■ HISTORY

Lithium was widely used in patent medicines and as a salt substitute for almost a century. In 1949, Cade, working in a remote Australian laboratory, reported on 19 psychiatric patients who received lithium. Even with this limited a sample, he was able to note an antimanic effect, but saw little impact on schizophrenic or on acutely depressed patients (1). There was a 20-year lag before it was fully approved in the United States. It is, by now, the cornerstone of treatment for acute mania and the prophylaxis of unipolar and bipolar patients. Recently, alternative agents have been investigated. Carbamazepine, marketed as an anticonvulsant, is now known to have a similar therapeutic profile, but different toxicities. Other anticonvulsants and calcium channel blockers are in the early stages of investigation.

## ■ LITHIUM

### *INDICATIONS*

#### MANIA

Lithium is clearly superior to placebo in acute mania. There is more of a question surrounding its role vis à vis antipsychotics, which are also helpful. Lithium's onset is slower, often not being fully apparent until 5 to 10 days after therapeutic levels are obtained (2). Antipsychotics work more quickly and are to be preferred when rapid behavioral control is necessary. Lithium has the advantage of creating less sedation. Those patients who are to be maintained on lithium can have it added, with the antipsychotic weaned once therapeutic levels are obtained. The usual "therapeutic" blood level is between 0.8 and 1.5 mEq/l. These figures are based on large populations of patients. Any individual can be outside this range and still do quite well. Doses should be decreased for maintenance, probably into the 0.6–0.8 mEq/l range.

Not all patients with mania should receive lithium. Maintenance treatment would not be justified for patients who cycle infrequently, since the potential for toxicity would outweigh the potential gain. The acute episode can often be managed with antipsychotics, unless lithium is to be used for maintenance. Patients with repeated seasonal illnesses may be able to manage by taking medication only at the time of year when they are vulnerable. Deciding on which patients with recurrent illnesses should be treated requires considerable wisdom. Table 1 summarizes some of the points that should be considered. This decision should be discussed in a forthright fashion with the patient and his or her family.

## DEPRESSION

There are conflicting data on lithium's role in the acute treatment of depression, although it is clearly not a first-line treatment (3). The more strongly bipolar the patient's or patient's family history, the more likely the patient is to respond to lithium while he or she is depressed. The support for lithium augmentation of antidepressants is clearer. There are suggestions that het-

TABLE 1. **Arguments For and Against Pharmacologic Treatment of Recurrent Illness**

| Arguments For Treatment |
| --- |
| Sudden deterioration without promontory warnings or insights |
| Marked behavioral dyscontrol with negative consequences |
| Strong family history |
| Absence of medication toxicity |
| Frequent cycling |
| **Arguments Against Treatment** |
| Good relationship among the physician, the patient, and the patient's family so that exacerbations will be reported early |
| Prominent early warning signs such as decreased sleep or increased energy |
| Illnesses that respond rapidly to treatment |
| Infrequent cycling |
| Exacerbations that do not include serious consequences |
| Toxic medications |

erocyclic antidepressants (HCAs) may accelerate cycling in bipolars. Lithium does not share this liability (4).

## PROPHYLACTICALLY, IN AFFECTIVE DISORDERS

It is in this area that lithium's effects are most dramatic. Lithium will decrease the number and severity of manic episodes and the number of depressive episodes. The intermorbid interval will be extended as well. Patients, even if fully compliant, may break through. Lithium's prevention is relative, not absolute. The National Institute of Mental Health's Consensus Development Conference on Pharmacologic Prevention of Recurrent Affective Disorders suggested that lithium was the drug of choice for bipolar patients or for patients with a bipolar family history. They felt there was equally strong support for HCAs and lithium in unipolar patients and that the choice should be based on whichever drug was most likely to enhance compliance. They suggested that the usual prophylactic level be in the 0.6–0.8 mEq/l range (5).

## SCHIZOPHRENIA, SCHIZOAFFECTIVE DISORDER

Approximately one-half of correctly diagnosed schizophrenic patients will show some improvement if lithium is added to their antipsychotic. The response rate is even higher if there is a strong affective component to the illness (6). Affective symptoms are most likely to respond, but there can be some improvement in core schizophrenic symptoms such as hallucinations, delusions, and formal thought disorder as well (7). In all, the response is less robust than that in affective disorder but is sufficient to justify a trial, usually adding lithium to antipsychotics, in treatment-refractory patients.

## ALCOHOLISM

A recent trial followed alcoholics for one year with conventional alcohol treatment combined with lithium or placebo. Lithium enhanced compliance. This is further discussed in Chapter 8.

## AGGRESSION

Lithium, when administered to prisoners lacking any psychiatric diagnosis, led to a significantly greater decrease in episodes of aggression as compared to placebo. Case reports have also supported its use with aggressive outbursts as the target in developmentally disabled and demented patients, but there are no controlled studies. Lithium, carbamazepine, and beta-blockers all have preliminary support, but there is no definitive treatment. This is discussed in Chapter 8.

## *TOXICITIES*

Most patients on lithium have some sort of toxicity. Generally, they are quite mild and well tolerated (8).

### INTOXICATION

Levels are a good guide to dosage, but should always be tempered with a physical examination. The signs of lithium intoxication are predictable and dose related. Considerable effort should be expended in educating patients as to the signs and symptoms associated with toxicity so that they may obtain help promptly. Table 2 includes the levels usually associated with particular toxicities.

A fine *tremor* is frequent, even at therapeutic doses. It rarely interferes with function, but some patients, such as musicians or surgeons, find it problematic. In these cases waiting for accommodation, reduction of dose, decreasing caffeine consumption, or low doses of a beta-blocker are all valid alternatives.

Lithium is a gastric irritant and should not be taken on an empty stomach. Even a few crackers prior to taking the medicine will be helpful. It should normally be given after meals. If *nausea*

TABLE 2. **Lithium Levels and Toxicity**

| |
|---|
| Early and benign |
| Tremor, nausea, polydipsia, polyuria |
| Levels at or above 2.0 mEq/1 |
| Diarrhea, vomiting, drowsiness, weakness, and decreased coordination |
| Levels above 2.5 mEq/1 |
| Ataxia, dizziness, tinnitus, blurred vision, cogwheeling, dysphasia, delirium, muscle twitching, hyperreflexia, fasciculations, focal neurologic signs, seizures, hyperpyrexia, coma |

does eventuate, then switching to an extended-release preparation is the best alternative.

There should not be exclusive reliance on the plasma level after an overdose because it may be only a poor reflection of what is going on in the brain. *Delirium* has persisted for days or weeks following peripheral normalization (9). Severe overdoses are managed with dialysis. More moderate cases are treated by osmotic diuresis, vigorous hydration, and alkalinized urine.

## ENDOCRINE

Hypothyroidism, by either laboratory or clinical parameters, occurs in 5% to 15% of long-term lithium patients. It is far more likely in women and often occurs during the first six months of therapy (10). This is not necessarily an indication to discontinue the lithium. Many patients are managed effectively with thyroid replacement. Since many of the symptoms of hypothyroidism mimic those of depression, it is always wise to check the thyroid function of a previously stable lithium patient who becomes depressed. More rarely, patients develop hyperthyroidism. *Thyroid abnormality* is more common in patients with previous history or family history of thyroid difficulties. Because of this it is wise to obtain baseline triiodothyronine, thyroxine, and thyroid-stimulating hormone (TSH) assays. The TSH should probably be monitored on a semiannual basis thereafter or whenever there is clinical suspicion of abnormality. Thyroid dysfunction should reverse with discontinuation of lithium.

Long-term lithium patients may develop statistical increases in calcium, ionized calcium, and parathyroid hormone levels (11). While it is decidedly unusual for this to be clinically evident, patients who develop ataxia, weakness, confusion, and lethargy while on lithium should have a calcium level drawn.

It is quite common to gain weight while on lithium. Multiple factors are probably involved. Lithium has a similar effect to insulin on carbohydrate metabolism. Patients may develop polydipsia and look to high-calorie liquids to quench their thirst. They are often coprescribed antidepressants and antipsychotics, which are also associated with *weight gain*. Patients, particularly those with a history of obesity, should be forewarned about this possibility and urged to exercise dietary caution.

## RENAL AND ELECTROLYTES

Lithium is primarily excreted through the kidneys. It is reabsorbed in the proximal tubule with sodium and water, but unlike sodium there is no further excretion in the distal nephron. If the body is experiencing a relative sodium deficiency it compensates by reabsorbing more sodium than normal proximally. Lithium is absorbed with it. Hence, the risk of lithium toxicity follows with hyponatremia. The import of this is that patients should be instructed to increase their salt intake in the face of exercise, fever, or other sources for increased diaphoresis. Sodium-wasting diuretics can be used with caution, but it should be realized that there will be an attendant increase in lithium levels.

It has long been noted that manic patients seem to require more lithium to achieve a given level. There is a suspicion that lithium clearance may be state dependent, but this has not been documented.

For many patients, lithium diminishes the response of adenylate cyclase to vasopressin and hence the ability to concentrate their urine. This is termed *nephrogenic diabetes insipidus* (NDI). NDI is related to cumulative lithium exposure. The result is that patients put out large quantities of dilute urine. The condition generally reverses after discontinuation of the drug. Significant polyuria is difficult for many patients to tolerate. If suspected, the clinician should monitor urine osmolality and a 24-hour urine volume. If these tests indicate the presence of NDI, then the alternatives are to discontinue lithium or to administer amiloride 5 mg b.i.d. along with the lithium (12).

More rarely, lithium patients can present with the nephrotic syndrome secondary to glomerular nephritis. This typically reverses with discontinuation of the lithium. Whether lithium causes diminution in the glomerular filtration rate (GFR) is less clear. Good studies require the use of a control group of affectively disordered patients not on lithium to ascertain if the drug itself is causing the change. It seems likely that there is a statistical, but small, *decrease in the GFR* with long-term lithium use, but significant decreases are rare (13). The decrease in the GFR is presumably secondary to tubulo-interstitial nephropathy (14). There is a suspicion that the effects relate to cumulative exposure and that therefore it would be prudent to maintain the lowest effective level. Serum creatinine and urinalysis should be monitored at baseline and every four to six months for patients on maintenance. If there is any evidence of proteinuria or of a rising creatinine, then more elaborate testing of renal functioning should be performed.

*Edema* is occasionally noted in patients on lithium. It is typically mild, transient, and localized to the pretibial area. It is not usually sufficient to warrant treatment, but does respond to diuretics, which should be used cautiously because of the risk of inducing lithium intoxication (15).

### CARDIOVASCULAR

One-quarter of patients on lithium will develop reversible, nonspecific *T-wave changes* similar to those seen with hypokalemia. Lithium replaces intracellular potassium; thus, the T-wave changes may reflect decreased intracellular potassium stores while serum potassium remains within normal limits. *Sinus node dysfunction* has been reported, but other arrythmias are rare (16).

### DERMATOLOGIC

*Psoriatic and acniform lesions* have been reported as well as various rashes. Lithium can also lead to *hair loss*.

### HEMATOPOIETIC

Lithium induces a reversible *leukocytosis* that remains so long as the drug is maintained. White counts of 13,000 to 15,000/ $mm^3$ are not unusual. The increase is usually in granulocytes and represents a step-up in the total body count, rather than margination. The effect is so predictable that lithium is being used as an adjunct to some chemotherapeutic programs. There are no other known hematologic effects.

### NEUROLOGIC

Many of the signs and symptoms discussed under intoxication are neurologic. Occasionally, patients develop *parkinsonian symptoms* on therapeutic doses of lithium. Cogwheeling is usually the most prominent symptom. It appears less responsive than neuroleptic-induced extrapyramidal syndromes to antiparkinsonian agents. There may be a subtle perceptual motor slowing, but there is no evidence for any cognitive effect secondary to the medication (17). There is continued debate about the effect of lithium on creativity. For a minority of patients, episodes of hypomania may well be connected with enhanced creativity. Such patients would associate lithium and euthymia with dulled creativity. For most, productivity is enhanced.

## *PHARMACOLOGY*

Lithium is a simple salt. There are several preparations available. Standard lithium carbonate is rapidly absorbed with peak blood levels obtained after about two hours. The elimination half-life for a single dose is about eight hours and in the 18- to 36-hour range once steady-state is obtained. It differs from most psychotropics in that it is not protein bound, does not have any metabolites, and is trapped in several organs including the kidney and thyroid. It is almost entirely excreted through the kidneys, with minor amounts in saliva, sweat, tears, and semen. Lithium levels could be monitored in any of these fluids, but custom dictates plasma levels, drawn approximately 12 hours after the last dose.

There are three different lithium preparations available in the United States: conventional lithium carbonate, available in 300 and 450 mg tablets and capsules; lithium citrate, a liquid with 5 ml equivalent to 300 mg; and extended-release lithium carbonate preparations.

Lithium citrate is used in patients who cannot swallow pills or are at high risk for cheeking medication and in geriatric patients where adjustment of the dose requires a dose increment less than 300 mg. Extended-release preparations are indicated where there is gastrointestinal toxicity or where b.i.d. dosing would enhance compliance. They are, however, more expensive.

Lithium is usually given either t.i.d. or q.i.d. Some advocate once-daily dosing with an extended-release preparation on the basis of the belief that the peak after absorption offers psychiatric protection and that the lower levels that would follow throughout the rest of the day would offer some protection to the kidney. There are not sufficient data at this point to justify this, but it is clear that many patients can do well with such a regimen. The major problem is gastric irritation with one large daily dose. If such a regimen is used, it should be realized that the 12-hour trough level will be higher than for the same total daily dose broken down more frequently.

Conventional lithium carbonate is usually begun with 300 mg t.i.d. for a normal-sized patient, then titrated by physical exam and blood levels to a target level. Dosage adjustments and levels can be done every three to five days.

Lithium discontinuation, even if done abruptly, is not associated with physical problems. The chief difficulty is the possibility of relapse.

## *LABORATORY MONITORING*

Table 3 contains one set of recommendations for routine monitoring of lithium. Once the dose is stabilized, the level will remain relatively constant, barring a change in the patient's physical or mental status. Until the medication regimen has stabilized, they will need to be drawn more frequently. Any elevation in the creatinine should be followed with a 24-hour creatinine clearance corrected for age and surface area.

## *INTERACTIONS*

Table 4 lists some of the better established interactions (18). At one time there was great concern about haloperidol. In retrospect, the reports seem to be variants of neuroleptic malignant syndrome. Haloperidol may have shown up simply because it is a commonly prescribed high-potency agent. The reaction is suffi-

TABLE 3. **Routine Laboratory Monitoring of Lithium**

| |
|---|
| At baseline |
| Triiodothyronine ($T_3$), thyroxine ($T_4$), thyroid-stimulating hormone |
| Serum creatinine |
| Urinalysis |
| Electrocardiogram, if cardiac risk factors exist |
| Every four to five months |
| Serum creatinine |
| Urinalysis |
| Thyroid-stimulating hormone |
| Lithium levels, once stable, can be checked every three months |

TABLE 4. **Lithium Drug Interactions**

| Drug | Effect |
|---|---|
| Antipsychotics | Coprescription, especially with high-potency agents, may increase the risk of neuroleptic malignant syndrome, although it is not clear if this is due to affective disorder or lithium. Somnambulism has also been reported. |
| Carbamazepine | Occasional case reports of neurotoxicity on the combination, although generally well tolerated. |
| Succinylcholine | Succinylcholine's effects have been prolonged. |
| Thiazides | Lithium clearance decreases. Lithium levels increase. As a rule of thumb: 500 mg of chlorothiazide will lead to a 40% increase in lithium level, 1 g 70% increase. |
| Nonsteroidal anti-inflamatory agents | Reduce lithium clearance and increase lithium levels. |

ciently rare that coprescription is quite justified, but an alert eye should be maintained. Because of the prolongation of succinylcholine, lithium should be discontinued for 48 hours prior to electroconvulsive therapy.

## ■ CARBAMAZEPINE

Carbamazepine is a tricyclic anticonvulsant commonly used for the treatment of complex partial and tonic-clonic seizures. It is being used increasingly in psychiatry, primarily as an alternative to lithium. Beneficial behavioral effects were noted in seizure patients who received the drug, but it was not apparent if this was secondary to replacing more toxic anticonvulsants or a direct psychotropic effect. Controlled trials now indicate that carbamazepine has a therapeutic profile very like lithium's; it is an effective agent for treating mania and for the prophylaxis of recurrent unipolar and bipolar disorder. It also has some (lesser) value in the treatment of depression. Preliminary data indicate that it may have some role in the treatment of aggression.

## *INDICATIONS*

### MANIA

When used in the usual anticonvulsant doses, carbamazepine demonstrates comparable efficacy to chlorpromazine and to lithium (19, 20). As with lithium, there may be a delay of 7 to 10 days before the full impact is apparent. Combination with an antipsychotic leads to greater effect than either drug alone (21). The likelihood of response seems as great whether or not the patient has an abnormal electroencephalogram. There are suggestions that patients who cycle rapidly (more than three episodes annually) are more likely to respond to carbamazepine, but this may be an artifact of the patients who were studied initially. It is clear that some patients may respond to carbamazepine but not lithium, and vice versa. The majority of patients will respond to both. Selection between the two is somewhat arbitrary. Lithium has frequent, generally mild side effects; carbamazepine rarely has toxicity, but it does carry the risk of one very unusual, very devastating problem—aplastic anemia.

### DEPRESSION

Of 35 depressed patients, many of them bipolar, one-third responded significantly, and 20 had at least mild improvement (22). These data are comparable to the impact of lithium.

### PROPHYLACTICALLY

Published data largely report on lithium-refractory patients, a rather skewed, difficult population, but even with this group there seems to be a positive impact of carbamazepine (23, 24). Carbamazepine's effects are relative and not absolute; there is a decrease in the frequency, severity, and duration of episodes, but breakthroughs can occur. There are not yet good data correlating dose or level and response. The usual custom is to aim for typical anticonvulsant blood levels of 8–12 $\mu$g/ml.

**VIOLENCE**

There is a growing, largely uncontrolled, literature looking at the impact of carbamazepine on violence among schizophrenic patients. All studies have looked at it as an adjunct to antipsychotics. The preliminary results are sufficiently exciting to warrant adjunctive use of carbamazepine for this indication. This topic is addressed in Chapter 8.

## *TOXICITY*

A skin rash is seen in 10% to 15% of patients. This is cause for discontinuation. Overly rapid initial escalations in dose are associated with decreased coordination, drowsiness, dizziness, slurred speech, and ataxia. These can be avoided by starting the drug slowly. As a tricyclic it shares all the advantages and liabilities possessed by other HCAs in terms of cardiac impact.

A transient leukopenia, with up to a 25% decrease in the white count, occurs in 10% of patients. A smaller percentage may have this persist as long as they are on the drug. This is not an indication for discontinuation. There have been several case reports of isolated thrombocytopenia as well. In the first 18 years that carbamazepine was marketed there were 20 patients who developed aplastic anemia. Frequently fatal, this disorder causes suppression of erythrocyte, granulocyte, and thrombocyte formation. A hematologist should be consulted immediately if suspicions are raised. The estimated prevalence is less than one per 50,000 patients exposed (25).

## *DOSAGE*

The usual practice is to aim for anticonvulsant levels of 6–12 μg/ml. It should be started with 200 mg b.i.d. with an increase to t.i.d. after three to five days. The first level should be drawn three to five days later. Levels should be drawn 12 hours after the last dose. The usual effective dose is between 600 and 1600 mg daily, divided b.i.d.–q.i.d. Cerebellar signs should lead to slower increments.

Carbamazepine induces the enzymes responsible for its own

metabolism. The effect of this is a predictable dip in level after three to four weeks of treatment. The physician should anticipate that an increase in dose will be necessary at that time so blood levels and clinical course should be closely monitored during this period.

## *LABORATORY MONITORING*

If the *Physician's Desk Reference* (PDR) recommendations were followed in full, the cost for a year's worth of laboratory tests would have been $2,161 in 1982 (25). Much of the testing mandated by the PDR seems unnecessary. The primary fear is of aplastic anemia, but its onset is sudden and unpredictable and it is unlikely that frequent complete blood counts would prevent it. Careful clinical assessment makes more sense. Patients should be instructed to monitor for petechiae, signs of infection, and anemia.

Discovery of a white count below 3,000/mm$^3$ or less than 1,500 granulocytes/mm$^3$ should lead to discontinuation of the carbamazepine. Table 5 contains suggestions for routine laboratory monitoring.

Hyponatremia can be associated with carbamazepine, so confusion or undue drowsiness are cause for a sequential multichannel autoanalyzer-6 (SMA-6).

TABLE 5. **Carbamazepine Laboratory Monitoring**

| |
|---|
| Complete blood count |
| At baseline and weekly for four weeks |
| Once stable every three months |
| With any sign of infection, anemia, or thrombocytopenia |
| Electrocardiogram |
| At baseline if at risk |
| Sequential multichannel autoanalyzer-6 |
| With symptoms suggestive of hyponatremia |
| Carbamazepine levels |
| Every week for four weeks |
| Every three months once stable |

### *INTERACTIONS*

There are several case reports of neurotoxicity with patients coprescribed lithium and carbamazepine. These are balanced by many more cases in which the combination was well tolerated. Whether there is any added benefit to using both drugs has not been documented, although individual patients unresponsive to both agents have responded to joint prescription. The more time-consuming, but prudent, course in a patient unresponsive to lithium is to discontinue it before beginning carbamazepine. If carbamazepine were to fail, then either coprescription, electroconvulsive therapy, or some of the alternative agents described in the next section could be considered.

The hepatic enzymes that metabolize carbamazepine are shared by a number of other agents. Cimetidine leads to increased carbamazepine levels, as does erythromycin, isoniazid, and propoxyphene. Carbamazepine has been suggested to decrease the effect of oral contraceptives, anticoagulants, phenytoin, primidone, valproate, and theophylline.

## ■ CHOOSING BETWEEN LITHIUM AND CARBAMAZEPINE

The data would seem to indicate comparable efficacy for lithium and carbamazepine. There are no reliable predictors of who will respond to which drug. Their chief difference is in terms of toxicity. A choice must be made between one agent with a high frequency of minor problems and another with a very low incidence of a very serious problem. This choice is best left to the clinician, the patient, and his or her family after they have been given as much information as possible.

## ■ ALTERNATIVE AGENTS IN BIPOLAR DISORDER

### *CLONAZEPAM*

Chouinard performed a randomized, double-blind, crossover trial comparing clonazepam and lithium in acute mania (26). Doses ranged from 4 to 16 mg for clonazepam and 900 to 2,100 mg for lithium. The results were comparable. There are no data comparing the two for maintenance.

### *VALPROATE*

Like clonazepam, valproate is used primarily for the treatment of absence seizures. It has been studied for prophylaxis of bipolar patients, for whom it seems to mute both depressive and manic episodes (27). Data for an acute antimanic effect are even more preliminary.

### *CALCIUM CHANNEL BLOCKERS*

There are several small studies of verapamil and one of diltiazem. Verapamil has been used in doses ranging from 160 to 480 mg in patients with acute mania. There are no controlled trials of maintenance. It has proved helpful in the limited numbers that have been studied (28).

## ■ REFERENCES


1. Cade JFJ: Lithium salts in the treatment of psychotic excitement. Med J Aust 1949; 2:349-352
2. Gershon S, Goodnick PJ: Lithium use in affective disorders. Psychiatric Annals 1981; 11:143-153
3. Jefferson JW, Greist JH, Ackerman DL, et al: Lithium Encyclopedia for Clinical Practice (second edition). Washington, DC, American Psychiatric Press, 1987
4. Wehr TA, Goodwin FK: Rapid cycling in manic-depressives induced by tricyclic antidepressants. Arch Gen Psychiatry 1979; 36:555-559
5. Consensus Development Panel: Mood disorders: pharmacologic prevention of recurrences. Am J Psychiatry 1985; 142:469-476
6. Delva NJ, Letemendia FJJ: Lithium treatment in schizophrenia and schizoaffective disorders. Br J Psychiatry 1982; 141:387-400
7. Zemlan FP, Hirschowitz J, Sautter FJ, et al: Impact of lithium therapy on core psychotic symptoms of schizophrenia. Br J Psychiatry 1984; 144:64-69
8. Jefferson JW, Greist JH: Lithium carbonate and carbamazepine side effects, in Hales RE, Frances AJ (eds): Psychiatry Update: American Psychiatric Association Annual Review (Volume 6). Washington, DC, American Psychiatric Press, 1987

9. DePaulo JR, Folstein MF, Correa EI: The course of delirium due to lithium intoxication. J Clin Psychiatry 1982; 43:447-449
10. Vestergaard P: Clinically important side effects of long term lithium treatment: a review. Acta Psychiatr Scand 1983; 67(supp):11-36
11. Franks RD, Dubovsky SL, Lifshitz M, et al: Long-term lithium carbonate therapy causes hyperparathyroidism. Arch Gen Psychiatry 1982; 39:1074-1077
12. Batlle DC, von Riotte AB, Gaviria M, et al: Amelioration of polyuria by amiloride in patients receiving long-term lithium therapy. N Engl J Med 1985; 312:408-414
13. Depaulo JR, Correa EI: Renal effects of lithium. International Drug Therapy Newsletter 1985; 20:13-15
14. Bendz H: Kidney function in lithium-treated patients: a literature survey. Acta Psychiatr Scand 1982; 68:303-324
15. Demers R, Heninger G: Pretibial edema and sodium retention during lithium carbonate treatment. JAMA 1970; 214:1845-1848
16. Guttmacher LB, Goldstein MG: Treatment of the cardiac impaired depressed patient: part two. Psychiatric Medicine (in press)
17. Squire LR, Judd LL, Janowsky DS, et al: Effects of lithium carbonate on memory and other cognitive functions. Am J Psychiatry 1980; 137:1042-1046
18. Jefferson JW, Greist JH, Baudhuin M: Lithium: interaction with other drugs. J Clin Psychopharmacol 1981; 1:124-134
19. Okuma T, Inanaga K, Otsuki S, et al: Comparison of the antimanic efficacy of carbamazepine and chlorpromazine: a double-blind controlled study. Psychopharmacology 1979; 66:211-217
20. Placidi GF, Lenzi A, Lazzerini F, et al: The comparative efficacy and safety of carbamazepine versus lithium: a randomized, double-blind 3-year trial in 83 patients. J Clin Psychiatry 1986; 47:490-494
21. Klein E, Bental E, Lerer B, et al: Carbamazepine and haloperidol v. placebo and haloperidol in excited psychoses. Arch Gen Psychiatry 1984; 41:165-170
22. Post RM, Uhde TW, Roy-Byrne PP, et al: Antidepressant effects of carbamazepine. Am J Psychiatry 1986; 143:29-34
23. Fawcett J, Kravitz HM: The long-term management of bipolar disorders with lithium, carbamazepine, and antidepressants. J Clin Psychiatry 1985; 46:58-60
24. Post RM, Uhde TW, Ballenger JC, et al: Prophylactic effect of carbamazepine in manic-depressive illness. Am J Psychiatry 1983; 140:1602-1604
25. Hart RG, Easton JD: Carbamazepine and hematological monitoring. Ann Neurol 1982; 11:309-312
26. Chouinard G, Young SN, Annable L: Antimanic effects of clonazepam. Biol Psychiatry 1983; 18:451-466

27. Puzynski S, Klosiewicz L: Valproic acid amide as a prophylactic agent in affective and schizoaffective disorders. Psychopharmacol Bull 1984; 20:151-159
28. Dubovsky SL: Calcium antagonists: a new class of psychiatric drugs? Psychiatric Annals 1986; 16:724-728

# ELECTROCONVULSIVE THERAPY



## ■ HISTORY

Other than malarial treatment for general paresis, there were no effective biologic treatments in psychiatry before the advent of convulsive therapies. A false premise—that epilepsy and schizophrenia could not coexist—led Meduna to attempt to induce seizures. Originally pharmacologic methods were used, but they were difficult to control. Finally, in 1938, Cerletti and Bini used electricity to trigger seizures. This turned out to be a far more predictable technique. Cerletti's original belief, that it was the seizure itself that had therapeutic value, not the method of induction, has stood the test of time.

The dramatic efficacy of electroconvulsive therapy (ECT), the absence of alternative treatments, and the fact that psychiatry now had a reimbursable procedure all led to a period of overuse. ECT was primitively administered without any anesthesia, oxygenation, or modification of the seizure. Little was known about limiting the memory impairment associated with the treatment. The inability to modify the peripheral manifestations of the seizure meant that fractures were common. Since then there have been dramatic improvements in the manner in which ECT is administered and increased understanding of what conditions the treatment is and is not helpful for. Unfortunately, these new perceptions have not been sufficiently shared with the public, whose only understanding of the treatment comes from such unfortunate portrayals as *One Flew Over the Cuckoo's Nest*. The result is that most patients enter into treatment far more apprehensive than they need to be.

The pendulum has probably swung too far in the opposite direction from the early period of indiscriminate overuse. ECT is increasingly reserved for patients in private and university settings. Veterans Administration and state hospital patients receive it far less frequently. Usage of ECT dropped from its maximum in the 1940s and 1950s in part because of the advent of effective pharmacologic interventions. The decline may now have leveled off. Simultaneously, there has been heightened academic interest. A new journal, *Convulsive Therapy*, has appeared and the number of scientific citations to this topic has increased dramatically (1).

## ■ EFFICACY

### *DEPRESSION*

Recently, the controlled trials comparing ECT with other agents in the treatment of depression were pooled (2). Table 1 summarizes their data.

The effects of ECT are clear. The surprisingly negative outcome for the monoamine oxidase inhibitor (MAOI) patients reflects one large study in which somewhat low doses were used, but the remaining data are about as expected for hospitalized patients.

It must be emphasized that these studies were only of acute treatment. ECT is the most efficacious therapy available for depression, but does very little to prevent recurrence. Since depression is often a relapsing disorder, patients should routinely have some sort of medication after their series. The analogy would be to treat a depressive episode with an antidepressant, but to then abruptly discontinue the medication once the episode had improved.

Use of ECT as opposed to heterocyclic antidepressants (HCAs) for major depression is associated with shorter hospital stays (3). Three-year follow-up data indicate lower mortality for ECT than for antidepressant-treated patients (4). Six-month fol-

TABLE 1. **Controlled Studies of Electroconvulsive Therapy (ECT) in Depression**

| | ECT | | Comparison Treatment | | Estimated % Advantage in Efficacy for ECT |
|---|---|---|---|---|---|
| | Responders | Nonresponders | Responders | Nonresponders | |
| ECT vs. Simulated ECT | 73 | 36 | 33 | 63 | 31 |
| ECT vs. Placebo | 138 | 22 | 69 | 86 | 41 |
| ECT vs. HCAs | 169 | 26 | 152 | 75 | 20 |
| ECT vs. MAOIs | 140 | 24 | 63 | 99 | 45 |

*Note*. HCA = heterocyclic antidepressant; MAOI = monoamine oxidase inhibitor From Janicak PG, Davis JM, Gibbons RD, et al: Efficacy of ECT: a meta-analysis. Am J Psychiatry 1985; 142:297-302.

low-up revealed fewer suicides and suicide attempts among patients treated with ECT than among patients treated with antidepressants (5).

Predictors of good response to ECT in depression are quite similar to those that augur well for antidepressants. Biologic signs are correlated with a positive response to both. The presence of mood-congruent psychotic features is associated with a better response to ECT than to antidepressants or antipsychotics alone, although antidepressants and antipsychotics combined do almost as well (6).

## *MANIA*

ECT is effective in the treatment of mania, but its use has largely been supplanted by antipsychotics and lithium. It is now typically reserved for patients who fail to respond to medication (see Table 2). A randomized prospective trial comparing lithium and ECT acutely in mania found the two treatments to be comparable. Both required several weeks for really significant impact. ECT patients who received lithium after their course were no more likely to relapse than were patients who received lithium throughout the trial. The most surprising result of this study was the ineffectiveness of unilateral, nondominant ECT. Originally, the trial included a unilateral arm, but this was dropped because of the ineffectiveness of the treatment (7). This is the only diagnosis to date in which unilateral technique has proved ineffective. Retrospective trials comparing ECT and antipsychotics in mania have found them to be comparable.

TABLE 2. **Indications for Electroconvulsive Therapy in Mania**

| |
|---|
| A manic episode refractory to three weeks of antipsychotic alone or antipsychotic and lithium |
| An episode of mania with excitement so severe as to pose a risk to the patient |
| Bilateral electroconvulsive therapy should be used |

## *SCHIZOPHRENIA*

From 1938, when ECT was discovered, until 1955, when chlorpromazine became available, ECT was the sole effective treatment for schizophrenia. Since then the use of ECT for this disorder has declined dramatically. It is now reserved for patients intolerant of antipsychotics or as a last resort for patients who failed to respond to several antipsychotics or antipsychotics and lithium. A recent review noted that ECT alone was ineffective in chronic schizophrenia and that its efficacy was inversely proportional to the duration of the illness. When used, ECT should be combined with continued antipsychotics, since the combination is more effective than ECT alone. Unilateral and bilateral ECT have comparable effect (8). When ECT is used, far more treatment is required: The usual norms are 6 to 12 treatments for depression and mania, but 12 to 20 for schizophrenia. What impact ECT has on the long-range outcome is still a largely unresearched question. The clinical impression is that patients tend to relapse after ECT is given and that the procedure, at best, buys a year or two of clinical improvement.

The predictors of good outcome are noted in Table 3. The more a patient's symptoms resemble schizoaffective disorder, the better the outcome. The more positive symptoms the patient has, the better the outcome as well. Some chronic patients lacking positive predictors do respond. They are rare and difficult to identify in advance, but a trial may be warranted, especially if it is understood that such treatment is a long shot.

TABLE 3. **Predictors of Positive Response to Electroconvulsive Therapy Among Patients with Schizophrenia**

| |
|---|
| Short duration of illness |
| Episodic course |
| Good functioning prior to illness |
| Significant paranoid, catatonic, or affective features |
| Positive symptoms |

## *DEPRESSIVE PSEUDODEMENTIA*

Depressed patients often present with significant cognitive impairment as one of the primary features of their illness. Demented patients often become depressed. There can be, then, a continuum between depression and dementia. It is often impossible to ascertain where a given patient falls along this spectrum without making an assumption of depression and attempting to treat. The alternatives for such a therapeutic/diagnostic trial are ECT and antidepressants. Either is justified, but ECT may be somewhat more rapid and is more definitive, given the greater efficacy (9). These patients should be treated with unilateral, nondominant technique since this is least likely to exacerbate their cognitive difficulties.

## *OTHER DISORDERS*

There are anecdotal reports supporting the use of ECT in a wide variety of other conditions, including obsessive–compulsive disorder, phobic disorders, substance abuse, chronic pain syndromes, etc. None is well supported scientifically.

# ■ PATTERN OF RESPONSE AND DURATION OF TREATMENT

Signs respond well before symptoms do. This means that others will notice the change before the patient does. Sleep and energy are valuable early indicators of response. Just as with antidepressant treatments, extra caution should be exercised during the period of recovery since the risk of suicide may actually increase before it gets better.

Treatments are typically given three times a week in the United States. The usual pattern is to see a brief antidepressant response after the second or third treatment, with gradually lengthening and more robust periods of remission as the series progresses. Figure 1 shows the prototypic pattern of response. There is, of course, considerable variation. Some patients may show nothing until the eighth treatment, then suddenly blossom. ECT should probably not be given up on until a patient shows no response after 10 to 12 treatments.

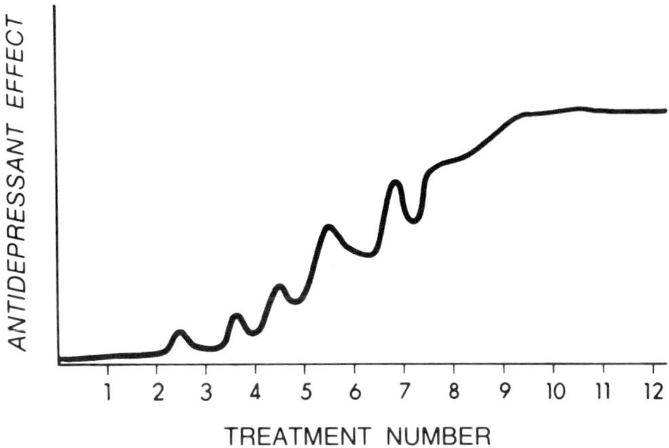


FIGURE 1. **Response to ECT.**

One of the most difficult questions surrounding ECT is that of how many treatments to give. Some physicians arbitrarily treat on the basis of diagnosis, such that all depressed patients receive eight treatments. Others wait until improvement has maximized, then add two more. This has been studied and there is no merit to adding the two treatments (10). The most logical approach is to continue to treat until the patient has either plateaued or had a decrease in the rate of improvement. This presupposes that treatment is not being limited by toxicity.

Diagnosis does afford some crude guidelines. Most depressed patients respond in 6 to 12 treatments, most manics in a like number, and typical schizophrenics in 12 to 20.

## ■ TOXICITY

There has never been much debate about the efficacy of ECT. The considerable controversy surrounding the treatment has largely centered around toxicity, especially the question of cognitive disturbance. Much of the debate has been based on emotion rather than science. The emotion should not be dismissed because it determines much of the climate surrounding the treatment. This had led to enactment of legislation in several states, such as California, so restricting ECT as to sharply curtail its use.

There is a very vocal minority of patients who feel ECT has severely damaged them. The majority of patients find ECT helpful and would repeat the experience. Only 18% of patients surveyed a year after ECT found it more upsetting than going to the dentist's office (11).

## *MORTALITY*

The mortality associated with modern ECT is approximately 4 per 100,000 treatments. This is less than the risk of barbiturate-induced anesthesia alone (12). What deaths there are are probably cardiac in origin. Modern technique has substantially lowered the mortality. ECT should be performed in a setting in which cardiac monitoring is available and resuscitation is possible. If adequately trained personnel are present, then the mortality would be even lower than the figure cited.

## *BRAIN DAMAGE*

ECT induces cerebral vasoconstriction. There is a transient increase in blood pressure and cerebral perfusion. Animals who are well ventilated do not experience cerebral anoxia. The older literature for both human and animal studies refers to punctate hemorrhages in brain, but it is likely that this represented agonal hypoxic change. There is a case report of an 89-year-old woman with bipolar illness who had 146 lifetime hospital admissions and in excess of 1,250 ECTs. After her death (unrelated to ECT) an autopsy was performed. Examination of the brain was entirely negative, except for changes consistent with aging (13).

There is generalized electroencephalogram (EEG) slowing associated with ECT. This generally reverts to normal within one month of the completion of a series, but rarely may persist for three months or more. Slowing is proportional to the number of treatments. There is no clear correlation between either clinical improvement or memory impairment and slowing (14).

Depression itself is frequently associated with cognitive impairment. This often makes it difficult to tease apart the effects of the treatment from the impact of the underlying disorder. Many

ECT patients experience an acute amnestic syndrome at the time of their treatment. There may be compromise in the ability to learn new information and difficulty in recalling data previously learned. These deficits are greatest for autobiographical information, especially for events that occurred around the time of the treatments.

The usual course is for the deficits to clear over the weeks after a series of treatments is concluded. Some patients report that they have persistent memory problems after ECT. Neuropsychological testing is not able to pick this up, which may speak more to the insensitivity of the testing than to the absence of the effect. One potential problem is the reliance on mean or modal values; perhaps there is an impact, but this is only for a small subgroup of patients who become lost among the larger body of patients who are not impaired (15). Freeman et al. attempted to address this by advertising in a local newspaper soliciting patients who felt that ECT had irreversibly impaired their memory (16). Patients were more cognitively impaired than a control group. When use of medication and ongoing psychopathology were controlled for, the complainers were statistically more impaired on 2 of 19 tests used. If, instead, a prospective methodology is used, focusing on the entire population of ECT patients, then the deficits tend to disappear, although it may take patients six months to fully return to their baseline (17).

For many patients memory improves dramatically as the depression resolves. One trial compared bilateral ECT with sham treatment in a depressed population. The simulated group had all aspects of the treatment save the passage of the electricity. Real, bilateral ECT acutely led to decreased concentration, short-term memory, and learning impairment, but improved remote memory. At six months no difference was apparent. Treatment-resistant patients, whether exposed to sham or real ECT, were significantly more likely to complain of memory impairment at six months (18).

Cognitive impairment associated with ECT has dramatically lessened as technique has improved. Electrode placement is a major predictor of memory disturbance. There is substantially more impairment among patients treated with bitemporal stimuli than among those treated with unilateral positioning over the hemisphere nondominant for speech. Newer machines feature a brief pulse wave form. Each stimulus consists of brief surges of electricity as opposed to the older sinusoidal current. The result is that far less electricity is required for seizure induction. The amount of current strongly correlates with confusion. Suprathreshold stimulation, or use of more than the minimal amount of electricity necessary to induce a seizure, will increase confusion. Patients with higher seizure thresholds, who are therefore exposed to more current, will experience more confusion.

Delirium is cumulative and proportional to the number of treatments in the series. Treatment more often than three times a week is associated with a denser delirium. Cognitive impairment can be minimized by using unilateral electrode placement, using the minimal amount of electricity necessary to induce a seizure, using a brief pulse machine, treating no more than three times a week, and giving the minimal effective number of treatments. There is debate as to whether some of these recommendations would impede efficacy. This is discussed in the section on technical issues.

## *NONCOGNITIVE NEUROLOGIC DYSFUNCTION*

We recently reviewed the data from our institution and found that the mean blood pressure recorded within one minute of the seizure was 201/116. This reverts to normal readings within minutes. The hypertensive reaction is secondary to the outpouring of catecholamines that accompanies any seizure. Despite this response, cerebrovascular accidents are not encountered. Apparently very brief, but very impressive, hypertensive surges are well tolerated.

"Tardive" seizures, or spontaneous seizures occurring after ECT, are occasionally seen, but they do not seem to occur more often than in the general population. ECT has even been used as a treatment for certain intractable epileptics.

Rarely, patients will have overly prolonged seizures with ECT. Seizures lasting longer than five minutes should be terminated with intravenous benzodiazepines or barbiturates. This is far more likely to occur with young patients or in patients who have an "irritable focus" (19).

Headaches are not uncommon for several hours after treatment. They typically respond to aspirin or acetaminophen. It is wise to give medication as soon as the gag reflex is intact for those patients who experience them on a repeated basis.

## *CARDIOVASCULAR*

We have recently completed a study of stable patients with high-risk cardiac histories, by virtue of past myocardial infarction, heart failure, or documented arrythmia, who received ECT. All patients were off of any medication that could affect rhythm for good or for ill. They all received 24-hour ambulatory electrocardiogram (EKG) monitoring for a day before and a day after treatment. Although we found significant rhythm disturbance, it was no greater after treatment than before.

A similarly high-risk population has been followed with serial creatinine kinase and serum glutamic oxaloacetic transaminase as markers of cardiac damage (20). No impact was seen. There is an increase in cardiac oxygen demand, associated with the increase in heart rate that is seen postictally (21). For this reason, it is probably wise to avoid ECT in the immediate period after myocardial infarction.

ECT may pose less risk than medication, particularly for those intolerant of antidepressants because of orthostasis, conduction disturbance, or arrythmia. ECT has the advantage of placing the patient at risk only for a brief period, during which it is possible to closely monitor the patient.

If ECT is to be performed in a high-risk population, then extra precautions should be exercised. Such patients should be cleared by a competent internist prior to treatment. IV access should be maintained until the patient is fully recovered. The EKG should be monitored for 15 minutes before and after each treatment. There should be staff present trained in cardiopulmonary resuscitation, and the requisite equipment for the treatment of cardiac emergencies should be immediately available. Serum electrolytes should be monitored between treatments for patients on diuretics or digoxin, since hypokalemia can be associated with prolonged succinylcholine effect and digoxin toxicity. Hypertensive patients may benefit from pretreatment with a beta-blocker or sublingual nifedipine.

### *MISCELLANEOUS*

Patients with *pseudocholinesterase deficiency* will have a very prolonged effect from succinylcholine. Such patients should be ventilated until spontaneous respirations return. At times intubation may be necessary. This disorder is genetically determined, so inquiry should be made as to either personal or familial history of anesthetic misadventures. It is sufficiently rare as to not justify routine testing.

*Myalgias* occur in about 5% of patients. They are rarely very bothersome and are helped by aspirin or acetaminophen.

## ■ TECHNIQUE

### *INFORMED CONSENT*

For legal, ethical, and clinical reasons, it is vital that a full explanation of the treatment take place. Well-educated patients are less anxious about and more tolerant of treatment. Our patients are visited separately by the psychiatrist, the nurse who directs the treatment service, and the anesthesiologist. We have found tours of the treatment area for patients and their families to be helpful in allaying apprehension. There is a videotape featuring Max Fink, one of the real authorities on ECT, explaining the treatment for patients and their families (available from Somatics, Inc., Unit 16, 910 Sherwood Drive, Lake Bluff, IL 60044). All such efforts at education are to be applauded.

The ECT service at the University of Rochester Medical Center has developed a detailed consent form that incorporates, but modifies, the information recommended by the American Psychiatric Association Task Force on ECT (22). It is reprinted as Table 4.

We were initially concerned that this amount of detail might be disquieting to patients, but have found the opposite to be the case.

The legal alternatives vary from state to state in terms of incompetent patients and ECT. One of the dilemmas is that patients with major depression are frequently imbued with profound hopelessness. They believe that nothing can help and extend this logic to include ECT. Other patients are convinced that

TABLE 4. **A Consent Form for Patients Being Treated with Electroconvulsive Therapy**

*CONSENT FORM*
*Electroconvulsive Therapy*

ECT has helped thousands of patients since 1938. It has been improved a great deal so that there are many fewer problems than there used to be.

Treatments are given in the morning before breakfast, about three times a week, by a psychiatrist, an anesthesiologist, and several nurses. While this is the usual schedule, your doctor may decide that some other schedule of treatments might be better for you.

Early in the morning of your treatment you will be given an injection or shot. It will make your mouth dry and will help to protect your heart throughout the treatment. In the treatment room you will be asked to lie down and you will be given oxygen through a face mask to help your breathing. Medicine which will make you feel sleepy will be given through a needle. You will also receive some other medicine, a muscle relaxant, through the same needle. As with any medicine, unexpected reactions might rarely occur. The treatment will be given while you are asleep. You should have no pain and will not remember the treatment. Two small round plates, called electrodes, will be held against your head and electricity passed through them. This will stimualte your brain and would ordinarily cause your body to shake and move strongly. The medicine you will have been given helps to protect you by almost completely getting rid of the shaking.

The treatment will take only a few minutes. You will awaken in the next room as if you were coming from a deep sleep. You may have some confusion as you are waking up. This usually goes away within a few hours. Nurses will stay with you until you are fully awake. Rarely, after the treatment some people may feel sick to their stomachs, have body aches, or headaches.

There are some other risks that could happen after the treatments. It may be hard to remember some things. You could have trouble remembering dates, the names of friends, or other facts. Normally this clears within four weeks after the last treatment. Very rarely aspiration leading to pneumonia can occur. Death is not very likely to happen. It has happened only once in every thirty thousand treatments.

The number of treatments you will have depends on how much they help you, but no more than 12 will be given without talking it over with you again. A second consent form would not be needed at that time if treatments were to continue.

*(cont.)*

TABLE 4. **A Consent Form for Patients Being Treated with Electroconvulsive Therapy** *(continued)*

You may stop the treatments at any time, but you will be asked to have as many as your doctor thinks you need. Feel free to ask your doctor or any of the ECT staff any questions that you may have.

I, ______________________________, have read about the treatments, and they have been explained to me by ______________ ______________________, who has also explained alternatives to ECT.

I agree to have treatments and anesthesia and understand that Dr. ______________________________ will be in charge of my treatments.

Signature ______________________ Date ______________

ECT will kill them, while at the same time being able to quote the data on the risk of mortality. These patients, if suicidal, may readily consent because they look forward to death. Informed consent is, then, a thorny issue.

## *PHYSICAL EVALUATION*

With modified ECT spinal films are unnecessary because spinal compression fractures are no longer seen. Routine laboratory studies should include an EKG, a chest film in those over age 35 or with history of cardiac or pulmonary disease or in smokers, a sequential multichannel autoanalysis-6 (SMA-6), and liver function tests. A thorough physical examination should be done. The only absolute contraindication to ECT is increased intracranial pressure, so focal neurological findings should prompt appropriate diagnostic studies to rule this out. Routine computerized tomographic scanning or EEGs in the absence of physical findings are not justified.

## *PRIOR TO TREATMENT*

Patients should have nothing to eat or drink after midnight in order to minimize any risk of aspiration.

Patients should ordinarily be pretreated with an anticholinergic in order to dry secretions, further minimizing the risk of aspiration, and to decrease the risk of arrhythmia. The usual dose is 0.4–1.2 mg IM 45 minutes before the treatment, or a similar dose IV just prior to the treatment. Patients who have difficulty with the anticholinergic impact may do somewhat better with glycopyrrolate 2 mg IM 45 minutes prior to treatment.

Patients should void prior to treatment to lessen the chance of embarrassing ictal incontinence.

## *THE TREATMENT TEAM AND THE TREATMENT*

ECT should be administered by a team consisting of a psychiatrist, an anesthesiologist, and a treatment room nurse. There will need to be another nurse to monitor recovery, if several patients are to be treated in succession.

### THE ANESTHESIOLOGIST

The anesthesiologist will gain IV access and administer a short-acting barbiturate and succinylcholine. The barbiturate is given so that the patient is asleep. If this were not the case, the patient might remember the onset of the inability to breathe induced by the succinylcholine, a terrifying experience. The barbiturate, typically either methohexital or thiopental, is anticonvulsant, so the minimal effective dose should be used. This may be titrated by the absence of the blink reflex, elicited by stroking the eyelash. Once the patient is fully asleep, succinylcholine can be given. Succinylcholine leads to paralysis, preventing the peripheral manifestations of the seizure, but also suppressing respiration. The patient therefore has to be ventilated. This can be done by either the anesthesiologist or the psychiatrist. Succinylcholine will cause fasciculations. Once they are complete in the calf muscles, it is safe to proceed with the treatment. Somewhat more reliable information is afforded by a nerve stimulator, a device that can be placed over the median nerve sending out a train of mild electrical charges that elicit movements in the hand. When these are no longer evident, the patient is ready for treatment.

## THE NURSE

The nurse in the treatment room should inflate a blood pressure cuff above systolic pressure on the right arm just prior to the injection of the succinylcholine and insert a rubber bite block prior to the stimulus. The cuff is intended to bar passage of significant amounts of succinylcholine into that arm. It is therefore possible to monitor largely unmodified seizure activity distal to the cuff. This poses no danger to the patient and, along with the EEG recording that should be obtained, offers confirmation that a seizure has taken place. If full modification occurs there may be no other evidence that this was the case. The cuff is placed on the right arm. Since the right side is controlled by the left cortex, right-sided motor activity after stimulation over the right hemisphere ensures that there was involvement of both motor cortices. Occasionally after unilateral stimulation, there is only contralateral activity. Such seizures are thought to be ineffective, and the patient should receive a second stimulus at a higher setting. The nurse's other, equally important, function is to offer support and reassurance to the patient.

## THE PSYCHIATRIST

The psychiatrist is usually in charge of ventilating the patient and delivering the stimulus. The patient is ventilated through the use of 100% oxygen delivered through a bag. The patient should be hyperventilated prior to the treatment since hypocarbia is associated with longer seizure duration, and this in turn correlates with better outcome. Ventilating can be resumed right after the stimulus, but now the rate should be slower as respiratory drive will be triggered by the $pCO_2$ returning to normal.

## THE TREATMENT

An EEG should be monitored. If a unilateral stimulus is used, then following the same logic as the blood pressure cuff, the recording electrodes should be placed over the contralateral hemisphere. With bilateral technique they can be placed frontally. The seizure should be at least 25 seconds clinically or 35 seconds by EEG. Seizure duration by EEG is always somewhat longer. Seizures shorter than 25 or 35 seconds are thought not to be antidepressant and restimulation should take place. The patient will be relatively refractory postictally so a higher setting will need to be used. Typical seizures are between 30 and 90 seconds.

Overly brief seizures are most likely with elderly patients. If this is the case, then a search for anticonvulsant medications, notably benzodiazepines, should be instituted. If found, they should be discontinued. Stimuli that are right on the seizure threshold may lead to incomplete seizures, so the setting should be increased slightly. If all else fails, then caffeine sodium benzoate, 500 mg, may be given IV prior to treatment (23). This proconvulsant should both lower seizure threshold and prolong seizure duration (23).

The ECT machine should deliver a brief pulse wave form because of the lesser amounts of electricity required. It should also have an impedance meter, attention to which prevents skin burns from developing. It should be capable of monitoring the EEG as confirmation that a seizure took place and that the duration was adequate.

Patients are typically asleep for two to three minutes, then awaken gradually. They should be turned on their side to prevent aspiration. Vital signs and consciousness should be monitored. They may return to their rooms once they are sufficiently awake as to be able to walk. They may find themselves somewhat sleepy for the remainder of the morning, but should be able to resume normal activities.

With improved technique, confusion has been minimized. This has allowed some patients to receive ECT on an outpatient basis. This is especially viable for patients who are receiving unilateral treatments and for those who have involved families who are able to drive them back and forth and stay with them for the morning of treatment

## *ELECTRODE PLACEMENT AND SETTINGS*

There is great debate in the field about the relative value of unilateral and bilateral stimuli. There is no quarrel about the associated cognitive impairment; acutely it is clearly less with unilateral, but this difference is not evident with long-term follow-up. The debate is whether unilateral works as well as or as rapidly as bilateral.

There have been over 30 trials comparing unilateral and bilateral ECT. Many have failed to detect a difference in efficacy, a similar number have shown a trend effect favoring bilateral, and a few have achieved statistical significance favoring bilateral. Much of the conflict reflects variability in diagnostic and outcome criteria as well as problems in technique.

Unilateral is somewhat more difficult to do well. The electrodes must be positioned more precisely and greater care must be taken to assure good contact between the electrodes and the scalp (24). The d'Elia position as shown in Figure 2 is preferred. Here one electrode is in a high centroparietal location, just to the right of the midline, and the other is placed over the right temple (25). If the electrode is not fastidiously positioned, there is the risk of establishing a current pathway that would bypass the motor cortex where much of the antidepressant impact might occur. The scalp must also be cleaned thoroughly with a saline solution just prior to treatment in order to assure good contact.

There are also data implying that unilateral ECT is less effective if the dose is very close to the seizure threshold (26). There is considerable variation in seizure threshold although certain predictors are known. It is higher for the elderly and increases across a series of treatments. Clinicians are faced with a dilemma: If unilateral is titrated down to the lowest setting that will induce a seizure, it is less effective; yet if pushed to a very high dose it will lose its advantage, which is lesser confusion, over bilateral. The usual compromise is to pick a low setting to begin with, but not to work assiduously at seeking the most minimal setting that will induce a seizure. If the initial setting does not lead to seizure activity, then a second, higher stimulus should be given.

The conflicting data are hard to reconcile, but some attempt at compromise can be arrived at. Two leaders in the field, Richard Abrams and Max Fink, attempted to develop guidelines (27). They suggest that patients start with unilateral treatment unless there is an emergency, as with acute suicidality or catatonia, or a history of past good response to bilateral. Manics should also always be treated bilaterally. If, after five to seven treatments there are no signs of response, then the patient should be switched

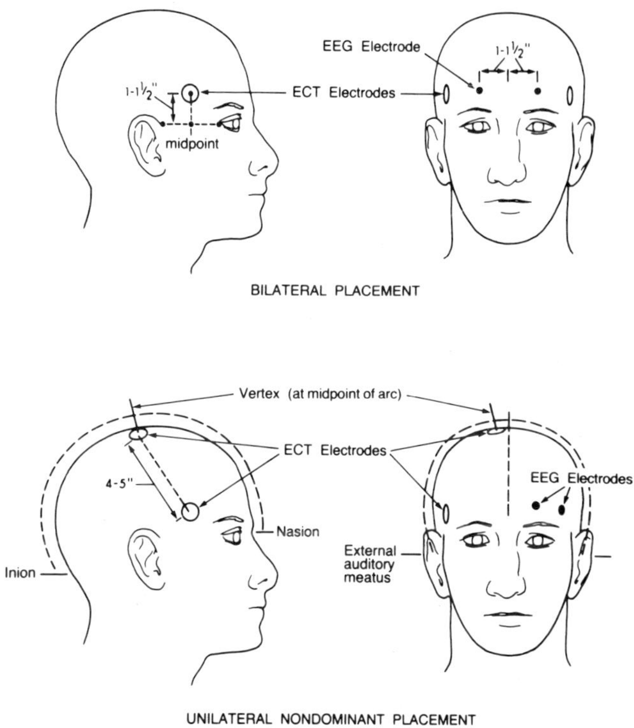


FIGURE 2. **Electrode Placement.**

to bilateral. Any unilateral treatments should be given at a low, but not minimal, setting.

## ■ ELECTROCONVULSIVE THERAPY AND MEDICATIONS

All patients should be off of benzodiazepines since they raise the seizure threshold, resulting in shorter, less effective seizures, more treatments, and larger doses of electricity. This would result in the patient's experiencing more confusion than is necessary (28).

MAOIs should be discontinued two weeks prior to ECT since they can lead to very prolonged apnea with succinylcholine (29). There is also concern that the catecholamines liberated by the seizure might lead to a hypertensive crisis.

Lithium also has the potential to prolong succinylcholine's effect and has been associated with more severe memory loss and atypical neurological findings (30). It should be discontinued 48 hours prior to ECT.

HCAs can be continued, but there is really no argument for doing so unless the patient will be going on the drug for maintenance. Even in such a case, it makes more sense to wait until the series is nearing an end before initiating treatment.

## ■ ELECTROCONVULSIVE THERAPY AND PHYSICAL ILLNESS

The only absolute contraindication to ECT is increased intracranial pressure. Space-occupying lesions in the brain, recent myocardial infarction, and some aneurysms are relative contraindications. Several conditions, including cardiac pacemakers and the need for anticoagulation, demand special cautions but can be managed safely. There are reports on the uneventful use of ECT in pregnancy.

Hypertensive patients may need to have their blood pressure brought under control prior to beginning treatment. Other patients who would be intolerant of the hypertensive surge postictally, such as patients who have had hypertensive cerebrovascular accidents, should be pretreated with beta-blockers or sublingual nifedipine.

Epileptic patients can be managed with ECT, but their anticonvulsants may need to be adjusted. The usual problem is that the drugs raise the seizure threshold sufficiently so that they are unable to seize. In such cases their medication needs to be decreased enough so that they are responsive to treatment, but not so much as to have spontaneous seizures. Some patients with seizure disorder enter into status epilepticus with treatment. This should be treated as any other ECT-induced status. An appropriate IV benzodiazepine like lorazepam should be kept available for such a situation.

## ■ MECHANISM OF ACTION

Chemical methods of seizure induction were effective as well, but were much more difficult to manage in a reproducible fashion and therefore are no longer used. The obvious conclusion from this is that it is the seizure, not the electricity or the method of induction, that matters. Modification of the seizure with retention of the treatment's efficacy argues that it is something about the central impact that is responsible.

There is no correlation between memory impairment and antidepressant effect. Many patients have full recovery without any cognitive impairment. The obvious conclusion, then, is that ECT works in some way other than causing patients to forget the source of their depression. Others have argued that ECT works by causing patients to feel as if they are being punished, thereby offering them a way to atone for their real or imagined sins. If this were the case, then we would expect sham ECT to be far more effective than it is.

Just as with antidepressants, there is no satisfactory single explanation for all the data, but several lines of argument may eventually prove to be of value. There are animal data to support the thesis that ECT acts by inhibition of kindling. The kindling model makes note of the fact that repeated subconvulsive stimuli will eventually lead to spontaneous seizure activity. ECT, like carbamazepine, is a potent inhibitor of kindling in the amygdala and may act by virtue of being anticonvulsant (31).

Like HCAs and MAOIs, ECT down-regulates the postsynaptic beta-receptor. This does not happen acutely, but only after animals have had daily treatments for a week. This property is shared by all effective biological treatments of depression (32).

## ■ REFERENCES

1. Fink M: Is ECT usage decreasing? Convulsive Therapy 1987; 3:171-173
2. Janicak PG, David JM, Gibbons RD, et al: Efficacy of ECT: a meta-analysis. Am J Psychiatry 1985; 142:297-302

3. Markowitz J, Brown R, Sweeney J, et al: Reduced length and cost of hospital stay for major depression in patients treated with ECT. Am J Psychiatry 1987; 144:1025-1029
4. Avery D, Winokur G: Mortality in depressed patients treated with electroconvulsive therapy and antidepressants. Arch Gen Psychiatry 1976; 33:1029-1037
5. Avery D, Winokur G: Suicide, attempted suicide, and relapse rates in depression. Arch Gen Psychiatry 1978; 35:749-763
6. Minter RE, Mandel MR: The treatment of psychotic major depressive disorder with drugs and electroconvulsive therapy. J Nerv Ment Dis 1979; 167:726-733
7. Small JG, Milstein V, Klapper MH, et al: Electroconvulsive therapy in the treatment of manic episodes. Ann NY Acad Sci 1986; 462:37-49
8. Small JG: Efficacy of electroconvulsive therapy in schizophrenia, mania, and other disorders, I: schizophrenia. Convulsive Therapy 1985; 1:263:270
9. Allen RM: Pseudodementia and ECT. Biol Psychiatry 1982; 17:1435-1443
10. Barton JL, Mehta S, Snaith RP: The prophylactic value of extra ECT in depressive illness. Acta Psychiatr Scand 1973; 49:386-392
11. Freeman CPL, Kendell RE: ECT, I: patients' experiences and attitudes. Br J Psychiatry 1980; 137:8-16
12. Fink M: Convulsive Therapy: Theory and Practice. New York, Raven, 1979
13. Lippmann S, Manshadi M, Wehry M, et al: 1,250 electroconvulsive treatments without evidence of brain injury. Br J Psychiatry 1985; 147:203-204
14. Weiner RD: The persistence of electroconvulsive therapy-induced changes in the electroencephalogram. J Nerv Ment Dis 1980; 168:224-228
15. Weiner RD: Does electroconvulsive therapy cause brain damage? The Behavioral and Brain Sciences 1984; 7:1-53
16. Freeman CPL, Weeks D, Kendall RE: ECT: II. Patients who complain. Br J Psychiatry 1980; 137:17-25
17. Taylor JR, Tompkins R, Demers R, et al: Electroconvulsive therapy and memory dysfunction: is there evidence for prolonged defects? Biol Psychiatry 1982; 17:1169-1193
18. Frith CD, Stevens M, Johnstone EC: Effects of ECT and depression on various aspects of memory. Br J Psychiatry 1983; 142:610-617
19. Guttmacher LB, Cretella H: The use of electroconvulsive therapy with three adolescents and one child. J Clin Psychiatry (in press)
20. Dec GW, Stern TA, Welch C: The effects of electroconvulsive therapy on serial electrocardiograms and serum cardiac enzyme values: a

prospective study of depressed hospitalized inpatients. JAMA 1985; 253:2525-2529

21. Mulgaokar GD, Dauchot PJ, Duffy JP, et al: Noninvasive assessment of electroconvulsive-induced changes in cardiac function. J Clin Psychiatry 1985; 46:479-482
22. Frankel FH (ed): Report No. 14 of the American Psychiatric Association Task Force on Convulsive Therapy. Washington, DC, American Psychiatric Association, 1978
23. Hinkle PE, Coffey CE, Weiner RD, et al: Use of caffeine to lengthen seizures in ECT. Am J Psychiatry 1987; 144:1143-1148
24. Weiner RD, Coffey CE: Minimizing therapeutic differences between bilateral and unilateral nondominant ECT. Convulsive Therapy 1986; 2:261-265
25. d'Elia G: Unilateral ECT. Acta Psychiatr Scand 1970; 215(supp):30-43
26. Sackheim HA, Decina P, Prohovnik I, et al: Dosage, seizure threshold, and the antidepressant efficacy of ECT. Ann NY Acad Sci 1986; 462:398-410
27. Abrams R, Fink M: The present status of unilateral ECT: some recommendations. J Affective Disord 1984; 7:245-247
28. Stromgren LS, Dahl J, Fieldborg N, et al: Factors influencing seizure duration and number of seizures applied in unilateral electroconvulsive therapy. Acta Psychiatr Scand 1980; 62:158-165
29. Marco LA, Randels PM: Succinylcholine drug interactions during electroconvulsive therapy. Biol Psychiatry 1979; 14:433-445
30. Small JG, Kellams JJ, Milstein V, et al: Complications with electroconvulsive treatment combined with lithium. Biol Psychiatry 1980; 15:103-112
31. Post RM, Putnam F, Uhde TW, et al: Electroconvulsive therapy as an anticonvulsant: implications for its mechanism of action in affective illness. Ann NY Acad Sci 1986; 462:376-388
32. Charney DS, Menkes DB, Heninger GB: Receptor sensitivity and the mechanism of action of antidepressant treatment. Arch Gen Psychiatry 1981; 38:1160-1180

# 6 AGENTS FOR THE TREATMENT OF GENERALIZED ANXIETY AND INSOMNIA

## ■ EPIDEMIOLOGY OF BENZODIAZEPINES

Benzodiazepines (BZDs) are the most widely prescribed class of psychotropics. It has been estimated that 500,000,000 people worldwide have had at least one BZD (1). During 1979, 11% of Americans between ages 18 and 79 had an anxiolytic; 1.6% of the population used these drugs every day during that year; 3.6% used them each day for a month or more. Long-term users were more likely to be female and elderly (2). Since 1979, American use has decreased by about one-third. The decrease probably reflects increasing awareness, by both physicians and the public, of the potentials for dependence and abuse. Given that the first BZD, chlordiazepoxide, was not marketed until 1960, the amount of use is still remarkable. Fortunately, the dramatic use of BZDs has been accompanied by a decrease in the prescription of barbiturates and meprobamate.

These drugs are prescribed much more often by primary care providers than by psychiatrists; only 10–15% of the patients described above had seen a mental health provider in the preceding year. Either the primary care givers are doing an excellent job of treating these patients, thereby obviating the need for a psychiatrist, or mental health providers are relatively more reluctant to prescribe them, possibly because of their awareness of alternative forms of therapy. Many anxious patients will respond to relaxation techniques, insight-oriented therapy, or other nonpharmacologic treatments. Given the potential toxicity of the BZDs, including dependence and cognitive difficulties, it is wise not to forget the therapeutic alternatives, especially if BZD use is to extend beyond a month or so. Unfortunately, there has been a tendency to line up in one of two camps with regard to BZDs. Klerman referred to these as representing a spectrum between "psychotropic hedonism and pharmacological Calvinism" (3). All too often this is based on the prescriber's value system rather than upon science.

All BZDs are anxiolytics, sedatives, anticonvulsants, and muscle relaxants. The choice of which indication is to be submitted to the Food and Drug Administration is partially a reflection of kinetics and partially of marketing strategy.

Basic pharmacology has been of more utility with the BZDs than other compounds. We understand the mechanism of action of the BZDs better than we do any other class of drugs. The kinetics very nicely predict the impact of these drugs.

This chapter addresses generalized anxiety disorder, but will not deal with obsessive–compulsive or panic disorders, which are mentioned in Chapter 8.

## ■ BENZODIAZEPINE EFFICACY IN GENERALIZED ANXIETY DISORDER

Estimates of moderate or marked response based on controlled trials are about 35% for placebo, 50% for barbiturates, and 75% for BZDs. Efficacy is highest for those with severe anxiety. Those who are only mildly anxious will often feel that the sedation outweighs any benefit. The presence of prominent somatic features is associated with good outcome. Depression, interpersonal difficulties, and obsessive–compulsive features are all prognostic of a poor response. A previous good result with anxiolytics augurs well, as does a positive expectation of benefit on behalf of the physician. The outcome after one week of treatment strongly correlates with more long-term results. If no improvement is seen after the first week, the patient is unlikely to respond further. Maximal improvement is generally evident by six weeks of treatment (4).

There is little in the way of controlled data on the use of BZDs in acute, situational anxiety. What data there are indicate that acute anxiety is very responsive to placebo. These patients have an expectation of improvement, and placebo or a BZD are therefore both associated with a good response. The difference between the two becomes apparent with more chronic anxiety.

## ■ DIFFERENTIAL DIAGNOSIS

The differential for anxiety is quite long and requires the clinician to pursue a careful review of systems. Table 1 summarizes some of the main items to be considered.

TABLE 1. **Physical Causes of Anxiety-Like Symptoms**

| Type of Cause | Specific Cause |
|---|---|
| Cardiovascular | Angina pectoris, arrhythmias, congestive heart failure, hypertension, hypovolemia, myocardial infarction, syncope (of multiple causes), valvular disease, vascular collapse (shock) |
| Dietary | Caffeinism, monosodium glutamate (Chinese restaurant syndrome), vitamin-deficiency diseases |
| Drug-related | Akathisia (secondary to antipsychotic drugs), anticholinergic toxicity, digitalis toxicity, hallucinogens, hypotensive agents, stimulants (amphetamines, cocaine, and related drugs), withdrawal syndromes (alcohol or sedative-hypnotics) |
| Hematologic | Anemias |
| Immunologic | Anaphylaxis, systemic lupus erythematosus |
| Metabolic | Hyperadrenalism (Cushing's disease), hyperkalemia, hyperthermia, hyperthyroidism, hypocalcemia, hypoglycemia, hyponatremia, hypothyroidism, menopause, porphyria (acute intermittent) |
| Neurologic | Encephalopathies (infectious, metabolic, and toxic), essential tremor, intracranial mass lesions, postconcussion syndrome, seizure disorders (especially of the temporal lobe), vertigo |
| Respiratory | Asthma, chronic obstructive pulmonary disease, pneumonia, pneumothorax, pulmonary edema, pulmonary embolism |
| Secreting tumors | Carcinoid, insulinoma, pheochromocytoma |

From Rosenbaum JF: Anxiety, in Outpatient Psychiatry: Diagnosis and Treatment. Edited by Lazare A. Baltimore, Williams & Wilkins, 1979. Reprinted with the permission of the publisher.

Several of the items in Table 1 should be emphasized. A very careful history of substance use and misuse should be elicited, with emphasis on stimulants (including caffeine) and alcohol. A physical exam with special attention toward thyroid dysfunction and pheochromocytoma is clearly indicated. It should be remembered that akathisia can present as a poorly localized sense of anxiety with patients receiving antipsychotics.

The primary psychiatric differential diagnosis includes atypical depression, panic disorder, phobias, obsessive–compulsive disorder, and any ego-dystonic perception.

It is also important to remember that all anxiety is not pathologic. Moderate amounts of anxiety often enhance performance. Treatment should be considered only when the anxiety bears little relationship to the stressor, when it is continuous, or when it restricts normal activities and functioning.

## ■ PHARMACOLOGY OF BENZODIAZEPINES

BZDs are rapidly absorbed from the gastrointestinal tract. Intramuscular (IM) absorption is quite variable and slower than that after oral ingestion. The one exception to this is lorazepam, which has dependable and rapid absorption after IM use (5). Midazolam, a very short-acting agent used to induce anesthesia or for invasive procedures, such as endoscopy, can be given either IM or intravenously (IV), but is not available for oral use.

### *METABOLISM*

All BZDs except lorazepam, oxazepam, and temazepam are metabolized chiefly by hepatic oxidation. This process occurs quite slowly and leads to many pharmacologically active metabolites. Oxidation slows with age and with hepatic insult, such as that induced by cirrhosis. It is also vulnerable to other drugs that can inhibit the enzymes—notably cimetidine, disulfiram, and estrogens. The remaining BZDs are metabolized by glucuronide conjugation. The result is that the drugs that are conjugated—lorazepam, oxazepam, and temazepam—are less vulnerable to drug interaction, have no psychoactive metabolites, are relatively shorter acting, and should be preferred in the elderly.

### *HALF-LIVES*

There is a marked difference in half-lives between single doses and steady-state kinetics. The drugs noted in Table 2 as having rapid onset are quite lipophilic. This facilitates rapid transit of the blood–brain barrier, but also results in a large volume of distribution. This in turn leads to a relatively brief duration of

TABLE 2. **Pharmacokinetics of Representative Benzodiazepines**

| Parent Generic Compound (Trade Name) and Half-Life | Clinically Significant Metabolites and Half-Lives | Approximate Dose Equivalence (mg) | Rapidity of Onset |
|---|---|---|---|
| Long Acting | | | |
| Chlordiazepoxide[a] (Librium), 5-30 hrs | Desmethylchlordiazepoxide, 5-30 hrs<br>Demoxepam<br>Desmethyldiazepam, 36-200 hrs | 10 | Intermediate |
| Diazepam[a] (Valium), 20-100 hrs | Desmethyldiazepam, 36-200 hrs | 5 | Fastest |
| Clorazepate[b] (Tranxene) | Desmethyldiazepam, 36-200 hrs | 7.5 | Fast |
| Flurazepam[a,b] (Dalmane) | Desalkylflurazepam, 40-250 hrs | 30 | Fast |
| Halazepam[b] (Paxipam) | Desmethyldiazepam, 36-200 hrs | 15 | |
| Prazepam[b] (Centrax) | Desmethyldiazepam, 36-200 hrs | 7.5 | |

| | | | |
|---|---|---|---|
| Intermediate | | | |
| Alprazolam (Xanax), 12-15 hrs | 4-OH-alprazolam<br>Alpha-OH-alprazolam<br>Desmethylalprazolam | 0.5 | Fast |
| Lorazepam[a] (Ativan), 10-20 hrs | — | 1 | Intermediate |
| Oxazepam (Serax), 4-15 hrs | — | 15 | Slow |
| Temazepam (Restoril), 8-22 hrs | — | 15 | Slow |
| Ultrashort | | | |
| Triazolam (Halcion), 3-5 hrs. | Alpha-hydroxytriazolam | 0.5 | Fast |

Modified from Greenblatt DJ, Shader RI, Divol M, et al: Benzodiazepines: a summary of pharmacokinetic properties. Br J Clin Pharmacol 1981; 11:11S-16S; and Rosenbaum JF: Current concepts in psychiatry: the drug treatment of anxiety. New Engl J Med 1982; 306:401-440.

[a] Available generically.

[b] Drug precursors that do not reach the systemic circulation in significant amounts without alteration.

effect for a single dose, since equilibration into the large fatty stores means that less drug is available acutely. This same process also means a very prolonged effect once steady state is reached since it takes a long time for the large volume of distribution to be cleared.

*Take note of the half-lives listed below.* Longer half-lives mean that accumulation is slow and extensive. It will take a long time to saturate the potential stores and to reach steady state. Washout of the drug will be similarly prolonged. Drugs with shorter half-lives will reach steady state much more rapidly, but accumulation will be much less. Ninety percent of steady state will be reached by the time four to five half-lives have been completed (6).

The kinetics noted above should determine which BZD is used for which purpose. An effective hypnotic should have a rapid onset of action; otherwise, the patient would have to either wait for several hours to feel the effect or plan well in advance on not being able to sleep. An as-needed (p.r.n.) anxiolytic should also have rapid onset. It should be noted that rapid onset is associated with a "rush" and increases the street value of an anxiolytic among drug abusers. Shorter durations of action are preferable in elderly patients for whom accumulation could be a problem. Also remember that all of the drugs listed are both anxiolytics and hypnotics, although they are marketed for only one indication. Lorazepam or alprazolam can be used as intermediate-duration hypnotics; flurazepam can be a long-acting anxiolytic.

## ■ INTERACTIONS

Cimetidine in particular, and disulfiram, estrogens, and alcohol to a lesser extent, have been known to inhibit the enzymes involved in oxidation, resulting in increased BZD levels for any given dose. The enzymes will be induced by cigarette smoking or heavy alcohol use, with lowered levels resulting. There is a report that coadministration of high doses of alprazolam and imipramine is associated with a significant increase in heterocyclic antidepressant (HCA) levels. HCA levels should be monitored if a BZD is also regularly taken.

The most significant interaction is that with alcohol and

other central nervous system (CNS) depressants. The effects are additive. It is very rare to see a successful BZD suicide that does not involve concomitant alcohol intake; coadministration turns a safe drug into a lethal combination. Patients should be cautioned not to operate heavy machinery or drive if they are taking BZDs and have any more than one drink.

## ■ TOXICITIES

### *ACUTE*

Early in treatment patients may be sedated, ataxic, or dizzy. These reactions are usually dose dependent and patients will accommodate to them with time.

### *OVERDOSE*

BZDs, unlike barbiturates, are remarkably safe drugs in terms of their potential as agents for suicide. Successful suicides almost always result from combination with other agents. The treatment of overdose is purely supportive, with the primary risk from respiratory depression.

### *ABUSE AND DEPENDENCE*

BZDs are less valued by drug abusers than barbiturates. Abuse is most common as part of a pattern of polysubstance abuse, particularly among methadone maintenance patients who use them to augment methadone's effects. Diazepam is generally preferred, probably because of its very rapid onset (7).

There has been long and heated debate about the potential for dependence associated with BZD use. While patients almost never need escalations in their doses, there is little doubt that there is potential for psychological dependence and that physical withdrawal is seen. Serious withdrawal syndromes are seen after high doses for prolonged periods, but even conventional doses may have rebound anxiety after cessation. Withdrawal is generally better tolerated with the BZDs than with barbiturates. The half-life of the drug predicts much of the severity of the withdrawal syndrome. Drugs with very long half-lives tend to taper themselves. Drugs with very short half-lives generally do not reach steady state. The most dangerous withdrawals are seen with drugs whose half-lives are in the range of 8 to 20 hours, such as meprobamate, secobarbital, alprazolam, and lorazepam (8).

There is an identical withdrawal syndrome seen after prolonged use of high doses of alcohol, barbiturates, and BZDs. There is cross-tolerance between these agents, so that a BZD can, for example, be used to manage alcohol withdrawal. The syndrome is characterized at various stages by anxiety, insomnia, tremor, irritability, headache, hyperacusis, muscle twitching, hypertension, tachycardia, hyperreflexia, nausea, fever, depersonalization, hallucinations, major motor seizures, and even death. The severity of the withdrawal correlates with the duration and amount of exposure. Symptoms tend to be minor with much less than four months of continuous treatment or with less than 30 mg of diazepam, or equivalent, daily. If patients have BZDs continuously for more than a month, then it is wise to taper the drug slowly, progressing no more than 10% per day. Reports have indicated that residua of BZD withdrawal may be apparent as long as six months after discontinuation.

Rickels has suggested that patients who are to be treated chronically with BZDs should have the smallest effective dose intermixed with periods off the drug. Such a program would prevent the development of physical dependence. Since the symptoms associated with the early phase of the withdrawal syndrome mimic those of anxiety, continuous use leads to a risk that patients will be maintained indefinitely on medication simply to counter the effects of discontinuing it (4).

## *COGNITIVE EFFECTS*

Short- and intermediate-acting BZDs have been associated with transient anterograde amnesia. Information is entered but not transferred from short-term to long-term memory stores. The cognitive impairment can be subtle but is sufficient that the physician should avoid triazolam and lorazepam, the drugs most frequently implicated, in treating cognitively compromised patients (9). Even cognitively intact patients exposed to typical doses of BZDs will show decrements in performance in tasks requiring attention, acquisition of new information, or such psychomotor skills as those required for simulated driving tests (10).

### *BEHAVIORAL EFFECTS*

Some patients, typically elderly and often with frontal lobe impairment, have BZDs prescribed for agitation and experience a paradoxical reaction with escalation of the target behaviors. This often leads to an increase in the BZD, further behavioral worsening, another escalation of dose, and so on. Remember that these drugs can make things worse as well as better (11).

Depression is also a well-known side effect of BZDs. It is more likely in those with history of affective disorder.

## ■ MECHANISM OF ACTION

The mechanism of action of the BZDs is better characterized than that of any other class of psychotropics. We know that there is a large receptor with specific recognition sites for the neurotransmitter, gamma aminobutyric acid, for barbiturates, and for BZDs. These act to open a channel for the chloride ion, which in turn alters the intracellular environment in the postsynaptic cell. The major importance of this is that very specific agonists and antagonists are being developed that may ultimately be of clinical utility and also further our understanding of the mechanism of anxiety.

## ■ DOSAGE

Anxiety should initially be treated on a p.r.n. basis. Treatment should attempt to address the underlying cause of the anxiety through the use of various psychotherapeutic techniques. If behavioral and psychologic interventions fail, it may, on rare occasions, prove necessary to move to the use of chronic BZDs. Such trait-anxiety patients should have therapy initiated with doses equivalent to diazepam 5 mg b.i.d. Adjustments should not be made until steady state has been reached, usually at four to five times the half-life. It would be highly unusual for a patient to require more than the equivalent of 40 mg of diazepam daily. Table 2 lists dose equivalents for various BZDs. Similar doses can be used for acute, situational anxiety when brief treatment is necessary.

## ■ NONBENZODIAZEPINE ANXIOLYTICS

### *ANTIHISTAMINES*

Antihistamines are really sedating, not anxiolytic, drugs, although hydroxyzine is occasionally used for this indication.

### *ANTIPSYCHOTICS*

Antipsychotics are reasonably effective anxiolytics, but their toxicity makes them an inappropriate choice for the treatment of anxiety, given the other alternatives.

### *BARBITURATES*

There is no longer any role for the use of barbiturates in the treatment of anxiety. Overdoses are far more lethal, withdrawal is far more dangerous, and their potential for abuse is higher. The only indication for continued use is as an anticonvulsant, as with phenobarbital, or as an anesthetic agent, such as thiopental or methohexital.

### *BETA-BLOCKERS*

Many of the symptoms associated with generalized anxiety disorder are mediated by the autonomic nervous system. Some British psychiatrists have distinguished between "somatic" and "psychic" anxiety. Controlled trials indicate that diazepam is helpful with both the physical and cognitive aspects of anxiety. Propranolol is helpful with the somatic manifestations, but does very little for the thoughts and feelings associated with the syndrome (12). There is one very interesting trial that found the combination to be more helpful than diazepam alone. Propranolol alone was less helpful than placebo in this chronically anxious population. Propranolol's augmentation of the BZD was most apparent when there was adrenergic blockade as manifested by a reduction in the resting pulse rate by 7.5 beats or more per minute (13).

There may be a role for beta-blockers in performance anxiety. A recent placebo-controlled trial studied beta-blockers with musicians suffering from stage fright. A single dose prior to the performance enhanced both the quality of the music and the musicians' experience of the recital (14). Similar outcomes have been reported for public speakers and surgeons. Some have questioned whether such use is ethically appropriate, especially given that beta-blockers are not benign drugs. Beta-blockers should not be given to asthmatic or diabetic patients or to those with congestive heart failure.

## *BUSPIRONE*

Buspirone (Buspar) is an azaspirodecanedione, structurally quite unique from other anxiolytics. Its primary advantage is its lack of toxicity. Unlike the BZDs, it is relatively nonsedating, does not alter the seizure threshold, does not interact with alcohol, and is not a muscle relaxant. It does not interact with the BZD receptor and therefore cannot be used for withdrawal from CNS depressants. It seems to have little liability for abuse.

Buspirone is well absorbed after oral use, with much of the drug lost to first-pass effect. It is metabolized via hepatic oxidation. Its kinetics are not much affected by aging. The reported half-life has ranged from 2 to 11 hours in various studies. Cirrhotics have a marked decrease in clearance, whereas renal failure has relatively little effect.

In chronic anxiety its effect has equaled diazepam's when they are compared on a mg-per-mg basis. The onset of either is not apparent until after one to two weeks of treatment. Trials have not looked at truly acute, situational use. It is not clear that buspirone would be effective on a p.r.n. basis. Typical dosing strategy is to begin with 5 mg t.i.d., advancing by 5 mg every three to four days until maximal benefit is reached. Doses in excess of 40 mg daily have at times been associated with dysphoria (15). Four percent of patients reported an increase in nervousness that was significantly greater than with placebo (16).

Buspirone was not marketed until 1987, so relatively little clinical data have accumulated.

## ■ TREATMENT OF INSOMNIA

One-third of Americans feel they have trouble sleeping; half of them consider the problem to be serious. One-tenth of that group, about 2% of the population, receive prescription hypnotics, and another 1% use over-the-counter hypnotics. A Consensus Development Conference, sponsored by the National Institute of Mental Health, emphasized that insomnia is a symptom of heterogeneous origin and that every attempt should be made to address the underlying cause. Patients should be treated with the smallest effective dose for the shortest clinically necessary period (17).

The Consensus Conference also suggested that a careful sleep history be obtained, including detailed questioning about sleep habits, use of alcohol and medication, and underlying medical or psychiatric disorders. Obese patients who are heavy snorers may have the sleep apnea syndrome, which will worsen markedly with BZDs. Careful inquiry of sleep partners may be helpful here. They felt that hypnotics were most appropriate for those experiencing transient insomnia of several days duration, such as hospital admissions; for travelers; and for those with short-term insomnia lasting as long as several weeks resulting from situational stress. They noted that insomnia lasting longer than that was psychiatric in origin from one-third to one-half of the time, even if substance abusers were not included in the psychiatric population.

They encouraged the use of nonpharmacologic treatment. Table 3 lists some nonpharmacologic approaches that may prove helpful. After these interventions have been exhausted, a short (less than one month) trial of hypnotics would be indicated.

They suggested use of a short-acting BZD as one alternative for transient insomniac patients. Patients with short-term insomnia respond particularly well to the measures outlined in Table 3, but may also require hypnotics. If there is not significant daytime anxiety, then a short-acting BZD is most appropriate. Use should be intermittent with a night off of medication after a good night's sleep. If long-term insomniacs have a negative workup and no underlying cause can be determined, then medication can be considered in combination with relaxation training and sleep hygiene techniques as outlined above. Their recommendation is for

TABLE 3. **Nonpharmacologic Sleep Aids**

1. Decrease caffeine
2. Eliminate alcohol and stimulant drugs
3. Exercise several hours before bedtime
4. Go to bed at the same time each night
5. Avoid using the bedroom for activities other than sleep
6. Stay out of bed if awake
7. Avoid daytime naps
8. Consider relaxation techniques

treatment approximately one night out of three, with the intervening nights available to assess progress. Intermittent use decreases the possibility of rebound insomnia, or a worsening of baseline insomnia seen after the discontinuation of hypnotics. It is more likely with long-term use and with long-half-life agents, but may exist even with one or two nights of a brief-duration BZD (18).

## *CHOOSING A HYPNOTIC*

Once again, the kinetics should dictate the choice of a particular agent. Temazepam is marketed as a hypnotic, but has a slow onset of action, generally leaving it as an inappropriate choice. Triazolam has a very rapid onset, but is of very short duration. It might be a better choice for a patient with initial insomnia than for another with midnight awakenings. Moreover, as noted above, there have been case reports of rebound anxiety on the day following very short-acting BZD hypnotics. Lorazepam, not marketed as a hypnotic, would be a logical choice for an elderly patient, because of its more rapid onset coupled with an absence of metabolites. Flurazepam would not be a good drug for elderly patients because of its very long half-life and potential for significant accumulation.

There is little reason to consider a non-BZD hypnotic, although many are available. Chloral hydrate is the alternative most often prescribed. The usual dose is 500 to 2000 mg.

## ■ REFERENCES

1. Ayd FJ: Social issues: misuse and abuse. Psychosomatics 1980; 21:10(suppl)21-25

2. Mellinger GD, Balter MB, Uhlenhuth EH: Prevalence and correlates of long-term regular use of anxiolytics. JAMA 1984; 251:375-379
3. Klerman GL: Psychotropic hedonism vs pharmacological Calvinism. Hastings Cent Rep 1973; 2:1-3
4. Rickels K, Schweizer EE: Current pharmacotherapy of anxiety and panic, in Psychopharmacology: The Third Generation of Progress. Edited by Meltzer HY. New York, Raven, 1987
5. Greenblatt DJ, Shader RI, Franke K, et al: Pharmacokinetics and bioavailability of intravenous, intramuscular, and oral lorazepam in humans. J Pharm Sci 1979; 68:57-63
6. Greenblatt DJ, Shader RI, Abernethy DR: Current status of benzodiazepines. N Engl J Med 1983; 309:354-358, 410-416
7. Griffiths RR, Sannerud CA: Abuse of and dependence on benzodiazepines and other anxiolytic/sedative drugs, in Psychopharmacology: The Third Generation of Progress. Edited by Meltzer HY. New York, Raven Press, 1987
8. Hollister LE: Clinical Pharmacology of Psychotherapeutic Drugs (second edition). New York, Churchill-Livingstone, 1983
9. Scharf MB, Saskin P, Fletcher K: Benzodiazepine-induced amnesia: clinical and laboratory findings. J Clin Psychiatry Monograph 1987; 5:14-17
10. Taylor JL, Tinklenberg JR: Cognitive impairment and benzodiazepines, in Psychopharmacology: The Third Generation of Progress. Edited by Meltzer HY. New York, Raven Press, 1987
11. Hall RCW, Zisook S: Paradoxical reactions to benzodiazepines. Br J Clin Pharmacol 1981; 11:91S-104S
12. Noyes R: Beta-blocking drugs and anxiety. Psychosomatics 1982; 23:155-170
13. Hallstrom C, Treasden I, Edwards JG, et al: Diazepam, propranolol, and their combination in the management of chronic anxiety. Br J Psychiatry 1981; 139:417-421
14. Brantigan CV, Brantigan TA, Joseph H: Effect of beta blockade and beta stimulation on stage fright. Am J Med 1982; 72:88-94
15. Griffith JD, Jasinski DR, Casten GP, et al: Investigation of the abuse potential of buspirone in alcohol-dependent patients. Am J Med 1986; 80(suppl 3B):30-35
16. Newton RE, Marunycz JD, Aldedice MT, et al: Review of the side effect profile of buspirone. Am J Med 1986; suppl 3B:17-21
17. Consensus Development Conference: Drugs and insomnia. Consensus Development Conference Summary 1983; 4(10)
18. Kales A, Scharf MB, Kales JD, et al: Rebound insomnia: a potential hazard following withdrawal of certain benzodiazepines. JAMA 1979; 241:1692-1695

# GERIATRIC PSYCHOPHARMACOLOGY

7

The elderly population is increasing rapidly. They pose a special challenge to psychiatrists for several reasons. The incidence of psychopathology increases in old age, but the presentation of psychiatric disorders may differ from that seen with younger patients. Older patients are often physically ill and exposed to a number of medications. The illnesses demand awareness of the impact of the physical difficulty on medications and vice versa. Differential diagnosis may become clouded by virtue of the somatic problems. This relationship between physical and mental illness often requires close collaboration between the internist or family physician and the psychiatrist. Age has predictable impact on kinetics by virtue of alterations in the organ systems involved in the various phases of drug disposition.

A number of generalizations about the elderly are made in this chapter. Realize, of course, that there are some 80-year-olds with the mind and body of a person 30 years their junior. Those patients should be treated as if they were 50.

In taking the history from an elderly patient it is important to get all the usual data, but several points need to be expanded on. The family history is taken, in part, to obtain genetic data. It now should include several generations of progenitors and of offspring. Elderly patients may have past psychiatric histories. A brief episode of hypomania 40 years before could have importance in assessing the risk posed by an antidepressant. Inquire carefully about drug exposure, including over-the-counter medications and alcohol as well as prescribed substances. The elderly are three times as likely to receive prescribed drugs as is the general population. Over-the-counter use is increased sevenfold (1). Find out about long-established personality traits by talking to family members. These are often exaggerated with the onset of dementia and disinhibition.

## ▪ PHARMACOKINETIC CHANGES WITH AGING

Table 1 summarizes the kinetic changes associated with aging (1–3). A review of some of the points made in Chapter 1 will further understanding of Table 1. Steady-state plasma levels increase with larger maintenance doses, absorption of higher percentages of the drug, longer half-lives, shorter dose intervals, and smaller volumes of distribution. Clearance increases with a larger volume of distribution and a shorter half-life. Clearance and steady-state level are inversely correlated. This is logical, since

TABLE 1. **Pharmacokinetics and Aging**

| Phase | Change | Effect |
|---|---|---|
| Absorption | Gastric pH increases<br>Decreased surface villi<br>Decreased gastric motility and delayed gastric emptying<br>Intestinal perfusion decreases | Little overall change<br>Absorption is slower, but just as complete |
| Distribution | Total body water and lean body mass decrease<br>Increased total body fat, more marked in women<br>Albumin decreases, gamma globulin increases, $alpha_1$ glycoprotein unchanged | Volume of distribution (Vd) increases for lipid-soluble drugs, decreases for water soluble drugs<br>The free, or unbound, percentage of albumin-bound drugs increases |
| Metabolism | Renal: Renal blood flow and glomerular filtration rates decrease<br>Hepatic: Decreased enzyme activity and perfusion | Decreased metabolism leads to prolonged half-lives, if Vd remains the same |
| Total body weight | Decreases | Think on a mg-per-kg basis |
| Receptor sensitivity | May increase | Greater effect |

From Thompson TL, Moran MG, Nies AS: Psychotropic drug use in the elderly. N Engl J Med 1983; 308:134-138; Greenblatt DJ, Divoll M, Abernethy DR, et al: Physiologic changes in old age: relation to altered drug disposition. J Am Geriatr Soc 1982; 30 (suppl):S6-S10; and Beattie BL, Sellers EM: Psychoactive drug use in the elderly: the pharmacokinetics. Psychosomatics 1979; 20:474-479.

the more rapidly a drug is cleared, the less of it is available. Clearance is more meaningful than the half-life. Lithium's half-life is prolonged in the elderly, but this is partially compensated for by the decreased volume of distribution.

The volume of distribution increases for all psychotropics with the exception of alcohol and lithium. The decrease in plasma proteins can lead to a higher percentage of unbound, free drug. Free drug crosses the blood–brain barrier and is psychoactive. Remember, though, that present plasma levels assay total drug and may not accurately reflect the amount of the drug that is available. Plasma proteins are also affected by malnutrition, so they may be compromised in an elderly impoverished or malabsorbing patient.

A decreased clearance and a prolonged half-life mean that it will take longer to reach steady state and to stop the effects of a drug. Practically, this means that the clinician working with older patients must move more slowly. The intervals between dose changes must be longer. Similarly, it will take longer to see if a drug will have impact. The smaller volume of distribution for lipid-soluble drugs means that smaller doses are required to have the same effect. In addition, there are indications that a change occurs in the sensitivity of the receptor for many drugs. Benzodiazepines (BZDs) and lithium will have a greater impact with the same blood level in an elderly patient. Heterocyclic antidepressants (HCAs) may not. The net effect of all this is that the wise clinician begins with lower doses with elderly patients, takes longer before making adjustments, and persists longer before declaring the drug a success or a failure.

## ■ ANTIPSYCHOTICS

Antipsychotics may be used for all the same reasons that are valid in younger patients. In addition, they may be used for management of agitation in some demented patients.

These are lipophilic compounds that are tightly bound to albumin and metabolized hepatically. The net effect is a large volume of distribution, a long half-life, and a low clearance. The evidence for increased dopamine receptor sensitivity is particularly compelling in patients with structural damage of the brain (4).

Even more than with young adults, toxicities must be taken into account when antipsychotics are chosen for aged patients. Elderly patients are more prone to parkinsonian side effects, with the curious exception of dystonias, which are decidedly rare. The incidence of akathisia increases with age. This is dose related and more likely with high-potency drugs. If these reactions develop, the treatment is to lower the dose or to switch to a lower potency agent. Anticholinergics should be avoided, because the elderly are especially prone to anticholinergic toxicity.

Be especially aware of the possibility of akathisia in a restrained patient. Demented patients tied into a gerichair due to agitation may be given an antipsychotic for the same indication. If akathisia results, the patient will become even more agitated because he or she will not be able to walk to discharge some of the anxiety. Prescription of more antipsychotic will only increase the toxicity and worsen the situation.

The alpha blocking property of the low-potency agents can lead to orthostasis, resulting in falls and broken hips. This risk increases with high-potency agents and with coprescription of HCAs.

Anticholinergic effects can exacerbate cognitive impairment and lead to delirium; constipation that causes impaction; urinary retention, especially in men with enlarged prostates; urinary tract infections; and visual blurring. These problems are most common with low-potency agents, especially thioridazine.

Phenothiazines, but not other antipsychotics, have been associated with agranulocytosis, especially in elderly women. This is most likely in the first two months. Because of this, elderly patients exposed to phenothiazines should have baseline complete blood counts drawn. A close eye should be maintained for the possibility of infection. Phenothiazines may also be associated with a poikilothermic reaction in the elderly.

The incidence of tardive dyskinesia increases with age, but there are a wide variety of senescent dyskinesias that can complicate differential diagnosis. A baseline AIMS exam should be performed (see chapter 2). Tardive dyskinesia is less likely to reverse among the elderly.

Patients should start with doses that are 10% to 25% of the usual younger adult doses, beginning with something like haloperidol 0.5 mg q.d.–b.i.d. and then adjusted from there. Intramuscular doses should be avoided to whatever extent possible, since the small muscle masses available may make them quite painful. Lower potency drugs are much more sedating, which may or may not be an advantage. The longer half-life in the elderly will beget accumulation and considerable daytime carryover even if taken at bedtime. The choice of an agent should take this into account as well as the question of whether the patient is at greater risk from parkinsonian-like symptoms or orthostasis and anticholinergic toxicities. As with all other agents in the elderly, doses should be adjusted less frequently.

## ■ ANTIDEPRESSANTS

Elderly patients have an increased incidence of depression compared to the general population. They are also more often prey to the many medical causes of depression, both idiopathic and iatrogenic. Because of this they should be very carefully reviewed for underlying physical disorder and medication status.

### *HETEROCYCLICS*

Heterocyclics are bound to alpha$_1$-glycoproteins, which are relatively less affected by aging than is albumin. The result is that the proportion of free drug should, in theory, be closer to that of young people. These drugs are metabolized hepatically. Patients given amitriptyline or imipramine, which are tertiary amine HCAs, will demethylate them, yielding nortriptyline and desipramine, secondary amine HCAs. This process is slowed in the elderly, resulting in relatively more of the parent compound. Table 3 in Chapter 3 establishes that the tertiary amine HCAs carry more risk because they are more potent antagonists of the cholinergic and alpha-adrenergic receptors. Since we want to avoid these toxicities in the elderly, it makes most sense to use the secondary metabolites. This choice is further supported by preliminary data for nortriptyline and desipramine indicating that the same blood levels associated with good outcome in younger patients probably operate in the elderly. Thus, nortriptyline levels between 50 and 150 ng/ml and desipramine levels greater than 125 ng/ml seem to correlate with antidepressant response.

The variability in the efficiency with which hepatic metabolism occurs in these patients leads to poor interindividual correlation between dose and level. Generally much lower doses should be used, with initial doses of 10 mg of nortriptyline or 20 mg of desipramine being appropriate, then increasing by a like amount, if tolerated, after five days. A level can then be checked a week later unless there is clear indication of response.

Almost all of the potential toxicities discussed in Chapter 3 will occur with greater frequency in the elderly population. Orthostasis is the most frequent dose-limiting effect. Anticholinergic toxicity, as discussed with antipsychotics, is even more of a problem with HCAs. The delay with cardiac conduction can be a major problem. The lack of anticholinergic impact or effect on conduction often leads to the choice of trazodone or monoamine oxidase inhibitors (MAOIs). Both suffer from problems with orthostasis. Trazodone also is very sedating and can further ventricular ectopy.

### *MONOAMINE OXIDASE INHIBITORS*

Since MAO activity increases with aging, there is basic science support for the utility of these drugs with older patients. Appropriate patients must be able to follow the diet or live in a setting that can guarantee adherence to the regimen. There are data supporting the efficacy of MAOIs in treatment-refractory geriatric patients. The absence of effect on cognition stands in contrast to HCAs and is particularly encouraging (5). Doses range from 15 to 75 mg for phenelzine and 10 to 40 mg for tranylcypromine.

## ■ LITHIUM

The indications for lithium are no different for older than for younger patients.

Elderly patients are often on drugs, such as digoxin, thiazides, or nonsteroidal anti-inflammatory agents, that interact with lithium. They will typically respond to both lower doses and lower levels than younger patients. Levels that would be well tolerated by younger patients may lead to toxicity in the old.

Serum creatinine, a relatively reliable screen for renal impairment in the young, is not helpful in the elderly. The loss of muscle that occurs with age means that a normal creatinine could occur at the same time there was serious renal damage. For this reason a 24-hour creatinine clearance should be obtained prior to beginning lithium and every six months thereafter.

The possibility of sinus mode dysfunction is greater with elderly patients, especially if they are on a digitalis preparation or a beta-blocker. Hypothyroidism is also more likely, as are parkinsonian symptoms. Lithium is a gastric irritant. An extended-release preparation may be better tolerated.

The decrease in the glomerular filtration rate and the decrease in the volume of distribution with aging result in appreciably higher levels for any given dose. Patients in their 70s will require 36% less lithium to achieve a given level than patients 50 years younger. This difference increases further with older patients (6). Moreover, elderly patients will respond to lower levels. Maintenance is usually accomplished with levels of 0.3 to 0.5, and acute treatment rarely requires levels greater than 0.8. Treatment is usually initiated with doses of 150 mg b.i.d. Dose increments and reevaluation can occur every five to seven days.

Several papers report on preliminary, but promising, trials of carbamazepine in geriatric patients. They have included patients with hyperactivity and/or emotional lability associated with dementia (7, 8).

## ■ ELECTROCONVULSIVE THERAPY

Electroconvulsive therapy is often given to the elderly. The indications and toxicities are covered in Chapter 5.

## ■ ANXIOLYTICS

The major pharmacokinetic change with age relating to BZDs is an increase in the volume of distribution for all compounds and a slowing in oxidative metabolism. Conjugative mechanisms are relatively unimpaired, so that the half-life for temazepam, oxazepam, and lorazepam changes very little, whereas the remaining BZDs are all significantly increased. This means that oxidatively cleared BZDs are much more likely to accumulate with the elderly. When this is combined with increased sensitivity to the drug, as appears to be the case, the dangers become apparent. A recent study assessed risk factors for hip fractures. As expected, HCAs and antipsychotics were implicated, presumably because of associated orthostasis and sedation. Long-acting, but not short-duration, BZDs were also found to increase the risk (9). This reflects the problem with accumulation.

Selection of a BZD should be based on rapidity of onset (which is a reflection of absorption and lipophilicity) and duration of effect. Short- and intermediate-half-life BZDs are less likely to accumulate. Those drugs that are metabolized by conjugation are to be preferred because of their greater safety. Long-half-life compounds, such as diazepam, chlordiazepoxide, or flurazepam, should not be used. The possibility of disinhibition with BZD use should be kept in mind. It is especially likely in cognitively compromised patients.

Oxazepam may be used in doses of 15 to 60 mg q.d. It is usually initiated with 15 mg q.d. or b.i.d., with titration no more rapidly than every three days. Lorazepam is given in doses ranging from 0.5 to 4.0 mg q.d., with the beginning dose 0.5 mg q.d. Both should be given b.i.d.–t.i.d. (4). These drugs may also be used as hypnotic agents, with some preference extended to lorazepam, which has more rapid onset.

Buspirone's kinetics are affected very little by aging, but there are few, if any, clinical studies with the elderly (10).

## ■ HYPNOTICS

Normal sleep architecture changes with aging. Phase advances are common, with the elderly retiring earlier and earlier. There are frequent midnight awakenings and compensatory daytime napping. Rapid eye movement (REM) sleep is distributed in shorter bursts and more evenly throughout the night. The very old and those suffering from Alzheimer's disease will have a reduction in the total amount of REM.

Sleep is further compromised by medical illness. Nocturnal angina may herald the onset of REM; chronic pain or paroxysmal nocturnal dyspnea may also awaken the patient. Institutionalized patients may be encouraged to sleep at a very early hour because of more limited staffing on evening shifts. Daytime naps may lead to difficulties with nighttime sleep. Dementia is associated with significant worsening of sleep. Sleep apnea increases markedly from both peripheral obstructive and central sources. Nocturnal myoclonus will manifest itself as episodic twitches of the legs that occur intermittently through the night (11).

The first stage of treatment should always be nonpharmacologic, with detail of a good sleep history. Daytime sleep habits, regularity of bedtime behavior, use of caffeine and alcohol, snoring, and nocturnal myoclonic jerks should all be inquired about. Good sleep hygiene habits should be encouraged (see Chapter 6, Table 3). Hypnotics should be avoided in those patients in whom sleep apnea is suspected. In the elderly, it is even more important to monitor daytime sequelae to hypnotic use. It should be remembered that no hypnotic should be prescribed on a nightly basis for an extended period. It is far more appropriate to use them 15 to 20 days out of the month, not allowing usage to extend beyond one or two months.

Unfortunately, there is a common belief that the antihistamine diphenhydramine (Benadryl) is a "mild" hypnotic. It is frequently prescribed on a nightly basis. It is also a potent anticholinergic, and patients are therefore exposed to anticholinergic toxicity. Nightly use also renders it ineffective for most patients within several weeks. Chloral hydrate is an old standard that is a more rational alternative to a BZD. It has a rapid onset, has a half-life of about eight hours, and poses fewer problems in terms of interactions. The effective dose ranges from 125 to 500 mg. It is a gastric irritant.

BZDs remain the cornerstone of hypnotic therapy with the aged. Long-acting hypnotics should never be used since the possibility of daytime carryover is too great. Triazolam is cleared by oxidative metabolism but has such a short half-life that accumulation is not a major problem. Its chief problem is its delayed onset. Temazepam has a somewhat longer half-life but is cleared by conjugation. The absence of metabolites means that it is even less likely to accumulate with chronic dosing than triazolam. Since the program of intermittent dosing outlined above would prevent accumulation of either, they would both be viable choices. If, for some reason, they were to be regularly prescribed, temazepam would be preferred. Temazepam is best begun with 15 mg, triazolam with 0.25 mg. Either could be doubled. Lorazepam 0.25 mg is yet another alternative.

## ■ TREATMENT OF AGITATION

Chapter 8 presents a more detailed discussion of differential diagnosis and the use of beta-blockers and carbamazepine in the treatment of agitation. In mixed populations of demented patients, antipsychotics have a modest effect in terms of treating agitation and aggression. This, limited as it is, is greater than that of BZDs (12). There are no trials comparing antipsychotics with beta-blockers or anticonvulsants. There is nothing to favor one antipsychotic over another, so prescription should be based along the lines mentioned previously.

## ■ TREATMENT OF DEMENTIA

There is no treatment for the cognitive aspects of Alzheimer's disease. These patients may become agitated or depressed or have difficulty sleeping. While we can address these behavioral concomitants, we cannot treat the primary disorder. Various nootropics, cerebral vasodilators, vitamins, and other nostrums have been advocated, but there is no real support for any such treatment. For now, we must await further research.

## ■ REFERENCES

1. Thompson TL, Moran MG, Nies AS: Psychotropic drug use in the elderly. N Engl J Med 1983; 308:134-138
2. Greenblatt DJ, Divoll M, Abernethy DR, et al: Physiologic changes in old age: relation to altered drug disposition. J Am Geriatr Soc 1982; 30 (suppl):S6-S10
3. Beattie BL, Sellers EM: Psychoactive drug use in the elderly: the pharmacokinetics. Psychosomatics 1979; 20:474-479
4. Salzman C: Clinical Geriatric Psychopharmacology, New York, McGraw-Hill, 1984
5. Georgatas A, Friedman E, McCarthy M, et al: Resistant geriatric depressions and therapeutic response to monoamine oxidase inhibitors. Biol Psychiatry 1983; 18:195-205
6. Jefferson JW, Greist JH, Ackerman DL, et al: Lithium Encyclopedia for Clinical Practice (second edition). Washington, DC, American Psychiatric Press, 1987
7. Chambers CA, Bain J, Rosbottom, et al: Carbamazepine in senile dementia and overactivity—a placebo controlled double blind trial. IRCS Med Sci 1982; 10:505-506

8. McAllister TW: Carbamazepine in mixed frontal lobe and psychiatric disorders. J Clin Psychiatry 1985; 46:393-394
9. Ray WA, Griffin MR, Schaffrer W, et al: Psychotropic drug use and the risk of hip fracture. N Engl J Med 1987; 316:363-369
10. Gammans RE, Mayol RF, Labudde JA: Metabolism and disposition of buspirone. Am J Med 1986; 80 (suppl 3B):41-51
11. Crook TH, Kupfer DJ, Hoch CC, et al: Treatment of sleep disorders in the elderly, in Psychopharmacology: The Third Generation of Progress. Edited by Meltzer HY. New York, Raven Press, 1987
12. Salzman C: Agitation in the elderly, in Psychopharmacology: The Third Generation of Progress. Edited by Meltzer HY. New York, Raven Press, 1987

# PSYCHOPHARMACOLOGIC TREATMENT OF SELECTED DISORDERS

8

## ■ AGGRESSION

Aggression may be a manifestation of disorders as diverse as paranoid schizophrenia, antisocial personality, and frontal lobe disinhibition. Whenever possible, the underlying cause should be treated, but there will be times when no clear etiology can be discerned or maximal treatment leaves violence untouched. For such patients, aggression may become a legitimate target in and of itself. The following discussion relates to psychiatric patients troubled by chronic violence.

A literature is now beginning to evolve focusing on violence as a target symptom. The patients studied have varied widely. Studies have at times been flawed by heterogeneous patient populations. A wide variety of drugs have been used.

### *ANTIPSYCHOTICS*

Antipsychotics are the drug of choice when violence is resultant from a thought disorder. Aggression and hostility in schizophrenic patients are among the target symptoms that are most likely to respond. Unfortunately, all such patients will not respond and other alternatives will need to be investigated. Patients who are not thought disordered are unlikely to respond in any fashion except nonspecifically to the sedation. This does not justify the potential toxicity. Neuroleptics should not ordinarily be used for this indication with nonpsychotic patients. An exception can be made for some demented patients. This is discussed in Chapter 7.

## *BENZODIAZEPINES*

There is little support for the use of anxiolytics in the treatment of chronic aggression. The primary benefit is sedation, which can be of considerable utility when confronted with an acutely agitated patient, but there are few data to support chronic use. If used, a wary eye should be maintained for behavioral disinhibition and worsening aggression.

## *BETA-BLOCKERS*

Most current research involves beta-blockers. This is in response to a series of promising, but uncontrolled, trials involving patients usually defined by a wide variety of organic impairments including cerebrovascular accidents, developmental disability, and Huntington's disease as well as schizophrenia. The one controlled trial involved aggressive inpatients suffering from various organic brain syndromes. They responded significantly better to propranolol than to placebo. The dose varied considerably, but the mean was 520 mg (1).

Guidelines for such use of beta-blockers have recently been published. Most literature has involved the use of propranolol, a lipophilic and therefore centrally active beta-blocker. Asthmatic and diabetic patients and those with congestive heart failure or unstable angina should not be given beta-blockers. Healthy patients can begin with 20 mg t.i.d. and increase by a similar amount every three days. Once there is evidence of beta blockade as manifested by a pulse below 50 or systolic pressure below 90, then no further increases are indicated. This will typically be at doses of 800 mg or less daily. The dose should be maintained for eight weeks or more in order to assess the impact of the medication. Concurrent alpha-blockers should be used with extreme caution due to the risk of hypotension. Beta-blockers should be discontinued gradually because of the risk of rebound hypertension. Tapering should be no more rapid than 60 mg daily with the last 60 mg being discontinued in 20 mg increments (2).

In summary, the use of beta-blockers in the treatment of aggression is promising but unproven. Patients with organic impairment are most likely to respond.

## *CARBAMAZEPINE AND OTHER ANTICONVULSANTS*

An early and uncontrolled literature supported the use of phenytoin (Dilantin) in the treatment of episodic dyscontrol. Controlled, double-blind trials failed to replicate the earlier claims. This should serve to caution in evaluating the more recent literature.

Carbamazepine seems to have somewhat more support, primarily in the treatment of violent schizophrenic patients refractory to antipsychotics. The original report was from Finland where a group of extraordinarily violent and chronic schizophrenic women had carbamazepine added to their antipsychotics. The response was quite dramatic, with significant decreases in violence, amount of antipsychotic prescribed, and degree of restriction required (3). A later report approaches being a controlled study. Luchins treated a group of similarly violent patients, all of whom had normal electroencephalograms (EEGs). When one patient developed a fatal agranulocytosis, the study was discontinued, allowing a comparison of the six weeks before the anticonvulsant, the six weeks before discontinuation, and the six weeks afterwards. Again, there was a significant effect favoring the drug. A second study by the same group showed similar results irrespective of EEG abnormality (4).

## *LITHIUM*

Cade's original description of lithium's psychotropic effects suggested antiaggressive efficacy. Curiously, the best studied population has been nonpsychiatrically defined prisoners. A double-blind, placebo-controlled study found that lithium maintained with levels in the 0.6–1.0 mEq/l range led to a significant decrease in major, aggressive infractions of prison discipline, but had only a minor effect on nonviolent transgressions (5). A similarly controlled study with aggressive developmentally disabled patients favored lithium over placebo (6). There have also been many positive case reports with both organically impaired and psychiatrically defined patients. Lithium appears to have considerable promise as an antiaggressive agent, but its target population, other than those with affective disorder, has yet to be defined.

In summary, lithium, carbamazepine, and beta-blockers appear to be best supported as agents for the treatment of aggression. The data are at best preliminary, and the appropriate target populations have not been specified. It is not yet clear that aggression can be treated separate from the underlying disorder. The primary disorder should always be treated first, with these agents reserved either to augment the response or for patients who are refractory to more conventional therapies.

## ■ ALCOHOLISM

### *DISULFIRAM*

Disulfiram (Antabuse) may be given to motivated alcoholic patients to decrease the likelihood of impulsive alcohol abuse. Within 12 hours of administration, disulfiram irreversibly inhibits aldehyde dehydrogenase, retarding the metabolism of alcohol and leading to increased levels of acetaldehyde if alcohol is consumed. *Restoration of aldehyde dehydrogenase activity requires six to seven days,* so alcoholics would need to plan a week in advance before drinking or risk a disulfiram–ethanol interaction. This is characterized by flushing, tachycardia, tachypnea, a sensation of warmth, palpitations, and shortness of breath in its milder form. If the alcohol exposure is higher, then it may progress on to nausea, vomiting, a severe headache, and loss of consciousness. Fatalities have been reported due to myocardial infarction and cerebrovascular accidents.

While many alcohol treatment workers believe that disulfiram has facilitated sobriety for significant numbers of patients, its efficacy has not been demonstrated in a controlled trial. If used, it should always be part of a larger treatment program (7).

The usual dose is 250 mg daily. Its use has been associated with exacerbation of thought disorder and depression, a not unexpected effect, since it also inhibits dopamine beta-hydroxylase, resulting in increased levels of dopamine and decreased levels of norepinephrine. It should not be prescribed for patients whose pulmonary or cardiovascular reserves are so limited that they have difficulty tolerating the alcohol–disulfiram interaction. The drug is metabolized via hepatic oxidation and should not be given to patients with advanced liver disease. The drug itself may be the cause of hepatotoxicity. It will interact with a number of drugs decreasing the metabolism of oral anticoagulants, benzodiazepines (BZDs) that are metabolized oxidatively, and phenytoin. It may make patients drowsy and should therefore be given at bedtime.

## *ANTIDEPRESSANTS*

Among alcohol abusers there appears to be some benefit derived from antidepressant treatment during the first three weeks of withdrawal, if depressive symptoms, anxiety, and physical discomfort are the targets After that time there is no greater benefit than that afforded by placebo. Interpretation of these data is complicated by the fact that almost all trials have suffered from low, possibly inadequate doses. Such skepticism is supported by the fact that because of hepatic enzyme induction, alcoholic patients require higher than normal doses to achieve therapeutic blood levels (8). In sum, it appears that antidepressants in relatively high doses may have a role in the first few weeks of abstinence, but there are not clear data supporting their use thereafter in an unselected population of alcoholic patients. Some alcoholic individuals do, of course, become depressed. They should be treated like anyone else who is depressed.

## *LITHIUM*

A somewhat more hopeful result was obtained from a recent, well-designed study with lithium. Patients were randomly assigned to placebo or lithium and followed for one year. They were also involved with Alcoholics Anonymous and an alcohol treatment program. Compliance itself, whether to lithium or placebo, was helpful, but chances of abstinence were furthered by having a lithium level of 0.4 mEq/l or higher. Patients were as likely to respond whether they were depressed or not (9). The authors caution that the study is too preliminary to justify routine use of lithium in alcoholism treatment, but further study is certainly warranted. The data appear somewhat conflicting and will probably remain so until we have better understanding of the relationship between alcoholism and affective disorder.

## ■ ALCOHOL WITHDRAWAL SYNDROME

Many different drugs have been advocated for the management of the alcohol withdrawal syndrome; all are based on the principle of finding something that is cross-tolerant with alcohol. It is then substituted for alcohol in sufficient amount to avoid withdrawal and tapered to avoid the discomfort and dangers experienced with abrupt discontinuation. In recent years BZDs have been the cornerstone of therapy. They have the advantage of substituting readily for alcohol, of offering sedation, of affording minimal respiratory depression, and of being anticonvulsant, thereby offering protection against "rum fits." This last quality makes BZDs preferred over antipsychotics.

Arguments can be made for various BZDs. Some prefer long-acting drugs such as chlordiazepoxide, with the idea of giving a large enough loading dose to suppress symptoms and then allowing the BZD to autotaper, thereby preventing later stages of withdrawal. While this approach is elegant in its simplicity, there are problems. There is great potential for accumulation, especially in patients who are prone to hepatic insufficiency. The ideal drug would not be affected by hepatic injury. Drugs cleared by conjugative metabolism would be preferred over those cleared oxidatively since they would be less affected by cirrhosis and since there would not be the problem of many metabolites and accumulation. Drugs that could be given orally, intravenously, or intramuscularly would offer considerably greater flexibility. Lorazepam comes closest to satisfying these criteria and has an intermediate half-life (10). Titration of dose to the patient's condition is vital, no matter which agent is used. Alcohol withdrawal is sufficiently predictable that the dose can be adjusted on the basis of the patient's vital signs and other physical findings. Tachycardia, hypertension, and hyperreflexia should be prevented while at the same time the patient is not allowed to become overly sedated. Because of the wide variability between patients, it is impossible to offer any absolute guidelines as to dose.

## ■ AMYTAL INTERVIEWS

Sodium amytal, a barbiturate, can be given intravenously to disinhibit patients. It has been recommended as an aid to interviewing mute or stuporous patients, for distinguishing between organic and functional illness, and as a therapeutic measure to facilitate abreaction surrounding traumatic events, recovery of function in conversion disorder, and memory in amnestics (11). The results are often dramatic, and the efficacy of the procedure was unchallenged until a placebo-controlled trial was designed. Placebo emerged every bit as effective (12). The reasons for this presumably reflect the very high expectations for the procedure, which is customarily surrounded by a great deal of drama and expectations of "truth serum." In addition, it allows for a concentrated clinical interview and much attention to the patient. In essence, it underscores the value of a good placebo.

## ■ COCAINE ABUSE

Preliminary data seem to indicate that antidepressants have a role in diminishing cocaine craving and depression after withdrawal. Trials to date have focused on desipramine, chosen because, like cocaine, it is an adrenergic drug (13). Anecdotal reports also find a role for imipramine. Monoamine oxidase inhibitors (MAOIs) have been advocated, but probably should be avoided since relapse with cocaine, a potent pressor, while on an MAOI could have dire consequences. Lithium, at least on an open, uncontrolled basis has seemed helpful to those cocaine abusers with history of bipolar disorder or cyclothymia. Pharmacotherapy should represent only one facet of a larger treatment program for cocaine abusers, just as for all other drug-dependent patients.

## ■ EATING DISORDERS

The distinction between anorexia nervosa and bulimia nervosa is underscored by the dramatic difference in response to pharmacotherapy. A recent study compared cyproheptadine, a serotonergic and histaminic antagonist, amitriptyline, and placebo. In a four-week trial cyproheptadine, with a maximal daily dose of 32 mg, was both antidepressant and associated with weight gain in the restrictive anorexic group, but was associated with deterioration in the bulimic group. It was remarkably well tolerated in a population that normally encounters many side effects (14). This is the first drug that has been of benefit in a well-designed, controlled trial with this population.

By contrast, many agents have been helpful with bulimic patients. Both heterocyclic antidepressants (HCAs) and MAOIs have assisted in decreasing the frequency of binges in bulimic patients. This appears to be true irrespective of whether the patients were also depressed at the time of treatment. Trials with doses below the usual antidepressant range have been less effective. There are no trials directly comparing MAOIs and HCAs. Most studies have been short term, although there are case reports with effect being maintained for several years. All studies have included pharmacotherapy as part of a larger, usually behavioral, treatment program.

## ■ OBSESSIVE COMPULSIVE DISORDER

In almost all disorders it is safe to generalize that all members of an effective class of drugs will be equally successful in treating the disorder. Obsessive compulsive disorder is the exception to the rule. There are strong data indicating that clomipramine is far more effective than any other medicine yet investigated, including other HCAs, MAOIs, antipsychotics, and anxiolytics. The response to clomipramine is as likely to occur whether the patient is depressed or not. At times there may be a dissociation between the antidepressant and antiobsessional effect. The latter is often considerably more delayed and may take as long as three months to reach maximal impact. Pharmacotherapy may be helpful with both obsessions and compulsions. Unfortunately, the response is imperfect: Only two-thirds of patients will have a moderate or marked response to clomipramine (15). Patients will, on occasion, respond to other agents. If clomipramine is unavailable, then treatment with a series of other antidepressant agents is warranted. Patients with compulsions will often respond very well to behavioral interventions.

## ■ PAIN

Many chronic pain patients are significantly depressed. This can be both secondary to the pain and a cause of the somatic distress itself. Antidepressants have analgesic properties irrespective of the presence of depression. The onset of action occurs earlier and at lower doses than the usual antidepressant effect (16). Both serotonergic and adrenergic HCAs and possibly MAOIs have been of benefit (17, 18). Treatment has been effective both as the only medication and adjunctively with more traditional analgesics. A wide variety of chronic pain syndromes have been studied. Since there are few data supporting a relationship between dose and response and since many patients respond to very low doses, it appears prudent to begin with very small amounts along the lines of 25 mg of imipramine or equivalent with the dose titrated from there.

## ■ PANIC DISORDER

Patients with panic disorder often suffer from two kinds of anxiety: the panic attacks themselves and anticipation of the panic. The second type, which may be quite devastating, will frequently beget agoraphobia and other avoidant behaviors. Most HCAs, MAOIs, and several atypical BZDs are of benefit in treating the panic component. Once medication has prevented panic attacks, then behavioral treatment is likely to be effective with the anticipatory aspect.

The controlled literature with HCAs has almost always cited imipramine. All trials have found it to be significantly better than placebo. A double-blind evaluation of trazodone found it to be without value, whereas imipramine- and alprazolam-treated patients did quite well in the same trial (19). The controlled trials of MAOIs have been as positive as those with imipramine. There is placebo-controlled support for alprazolam and a considerable, uncontrolled, positive literature about clonazepam among the BZDs. Trials of other BZDs have been either negative or equivocal.

Although MAOIs are effective, they are infrequently used as a first-line drug for this indication because there are other equally effective alternatives that do not require adherence to a diet. The choice, then, comes down to an HCA, usually imipramine, or alprazolam or clonazepam. The BZDs have the advantage of having some minor effect on the anticipatory component and of being somewhat less difficult to begin. Imipramine is difficult to initiate, but does not pose a problem in terms of withdrawal.

Panic-disordered patients are exquisitely aware of their bodies and are desperately searching for an explanation for their dysphoric somatic sensations. Some studies have found the majority of patients unable to tolerate maximal doses of placebo due to side effects. HCAs cause some of the sensations usually connected with anxiety—tachycardia, dry mouth, and lightheadedness. Unless this problem is anticipated and discussed in advance, many patients will have a difficult time in tolerating the initial stages of imipramine. Data are conflicting on dose and response, but it looks as if patients do best if full antidepressant doses are used. Because of the difficulty with compliance and initiating the medicine, I customarily start with a lower dose of 25 mg and advance more slowly than with patients suffering from depression. The same latency seen in treating depression occurs since most patients do not respond before two weeks.

Alprazolam is better tolerated in the beginning. Patients will require substantially higher doses than they would for generalized anxiety disorder. Doses are usually in the 4 to 9 mg q.d. range. The major liability is in terms of discontinuation. Panic disorder tends to be a chronic, unremittent disorder. Some patients do have spontaneous recoveries, nonetheless, so it is wise to slowly taper the drug every six months. Occasionally, patients can do without any medication. More often they are able to manage with a lower dose. Alprazolam, with its short to intermediate half-life, is extremely difficult to discontinue. Clonazepam (Klonopin), another BZD, is normally used as an anticonvulsant. It has a longer half-life and poses less of a problem in terms of discontinuation. The literature is entirely uncontrolled, but some centers are using substantially lower doses, along the lines of 1.5 to 3 mg q.d., with success.

## ■ PERSONALITY DISORDERS

Good clinical trials have been rare with patients largely because of the diagnostic heterogeneity of patients subsumed under these labels. Recently some better studies have begun to emerge. A series of trials from the National Institute of Mental Health indicate that carbamazepine is helpful with the behavioral dyscontrol and impulsivity sometimes seen with patients suffering from borderline personality disorder (20). Alprazolam, on the other hand, seems associated with disinhibition and worsening of this problem (21). Low doses (mean 7.24 mg q.d.) of haloperidol were helpful with borderline inpatients in addressing hostility, paranoia, anxiety, and depression. Amitryptiline was no better than placebo and was associated with worsening in some patients (22). Antipsychotics would seem to have a role for thought disordered, and perhaps even depressed, borderline patients. Carbamazepine seems to be helpful for impulsive borderlines.

## ■ PREGNANCY AND PSYCHOPHARMACOLOGY

Proving the null hypothesis, in this case that a drug does not cause problems for the fetus, is impossible. There are a number of methodologic problems, mostly relating to sample size. Malformations are rare events. To say that a drug does not double the chance of malformation may require a sample of 50,000. Moreover, an appropriate control group would be of parents who are suffering from the same disorder but are not receiving medication for it. Otherwise, it would be possible that the illness itself might increase the chance of malformation. Many mechanisms could be postulated, ranging from a common genetic locus to psychiatric disorder leading to inadequate antepartum diet and care. Things become even more complicated if we talk of anything other than congenital anomaly or miscarriage. Recently there has been interest in the idea of behavioral teratogens, or insults such as drug exposure during pregnancy manifesting later as behavioral disturbance in the child.

The only reliable system for implicating a drug is in picking up an unusually high incidence of an otherwise rare anomaly and then being able to trace back to a common drug exposure in a number of mothers. This was the case with the hypnotic thalidomide, which led to phocomelia, and has been seen again with lithium, which is associated with an otherwise rare cardiac abnormality, Ebstein's anomaly, when taken during the first trimester. It has been estimated that the chance of Ebstein's anomaly in lithium offspring is one in one thousand. The parents and their physician are left in the position of having to balance that against the potential risk of untreated psychiatric disorder, about which even less is known.

Unfortunately, those factors predictive of crossing the blood brain–barrier are the same ones that predict crossing the placenta. The time of greatest risk for the fetus is during the period of organogenesis from days 17 to 70 of the pregnancy. Some women will not be aware of their pregnancy by day 17. Drugs that accumulate, as many psychotropics do, will continue to exert their effect for a substantial period after discontinuation. These facts mean that the possibility of pregnancy should be discussed in advance and good contraceptive practices should be encouraged. Use of psychotropics during the first trimester should be minimized to whatever extent possible.

Drugs taken later in pregnancy may affect the fetus through postpartum respiratory depression, neonatal jaundice, or hyperbilirubinemia. They might also induce fetal distress and premature deliveries. There is also the possibility of creating a withdrawal syndrome in the newborn.

## *ANTIPSYCHOTICS*

Dopamine blockade can induce menstrual irregularity. Patients need to be told that this is not a reliable form of contraception.

Offspring of schizophrenic individuals have an increased incidence of congenital anomalies compared to the general population, but the poor outcome appears to correlate more highly with severity of illness and chronicity than with medication status (23). No particular anomaly has been associated with the use of antipsychotics. Neuroleptic use late in pregnancy can lead to extrapyramidal syndromes and sedation in the neonate. Hyperbilirubinemia, neonatal jaundice, and hepatic enzyme induction have also been reported (24).

## *LITHIUM*

As previously discussed, the incidence of Ebstein's anomaly of the tricuspid valve has been estimated as 0.1% in the children of mothers exposed to lithium (25). First-trimester use should therefore be avoided. If pregnancy is being considered, it might be wiser to switch to carbamazepine or a neuroleptic for prophylaxis or to consider the option of discontinuing medication completely. An acute manic episode during the first trimester should be managed with one of the agents above or with electroconvulsive therapy (ECT).

Pregnancy leads to an increase in the glomerular filtration rate, so lithium doses may need to increase if used during the last two trimesters. There is often a sudden decrease in lithium clearance in the 24 hours prior to labor, leaving the possibility of sudden lithium toxicity. The difficulty is that it is impossible to know when labor will occur. Lithium should be very closely monitored during this period. Lithium offspring have been reported as floppy and lethargic. There have also been reports of reversible, neonatal goiter. Decisions on management of the bipolar pregnant patient should integrate the data that indicate a greatly increased risk of affective disorder in the postpartum period among these patients.

## *CARBAMAZEPINE*

Carbamazepine is the fourth most commonly prescribed anticonvulsant and has been available for the past 20 years. Even with this widespread use in neurology, there have not been reports of specific anomalies. It is generally considered the safest of the anticonvulsants.

## *ELECTROCONVULSIVE THERAPY*

The literature includes several dozen patients who have received ECT in pregnancy. Most were in the second or third trimester. No problems have been reported. The obstetrician should become a member of the treatment team and fetal monitoring should be performed with advanced pregnancies. While there is not a great deal of data, it appears that ECT might pose a reasonable alternative for some psychotic patients.

## *ANTIDEPRESSANTS*

There is a paucity of data on these drugs, but the HCAs appear to be quite safe in terms of malformation. MAOIs are prescribed sufficiently rarely that it is not possible to offer even tentative epidemiologically based conclusions. Neonatal withdrawal has been reported with HCAs with dyspnea, difficulty in feeding, irritability, and urinary retention. Ideally, the drug should be withdrawn or the dose decreased prior to term.

## *BENZODIAZEPINES*

There has been debate as to whether first-trimester use is associated with cleft palates. More recent data indicate that it probably is not. There are clear data on a BZD neonatal withdrawal syndrome. The maternal liver is better able to metabolize BZDs than is a neonate's, so it is probably preferable to taper the drug in utero rather than after birth (26). Since BZD use is usually less emergent than other psychotropics, it would be wise to avoid their use.

## *BREAST-FEEDING*

Most psychotropics are excreted in breast milk. The amount varies and we are typically unclear on how much of a given drug an infant can tolerate. Guidelines are generally based on supposition, although there are occasional reports of toxicity, which can guide us more effectively.

Antipsychotics are passed into breast milk, but in low concentration. There is not any evidence of a clear effect on the infant. Lithium can appear in breast milk at half the concentration seen in maternal plasma. Lithium toxicity has been reported in breast-fed children, especially when dehydrated. It appears that both HCAs and MAOIs are excreted in such low amounts as to be safe for nursing mothers. Lethargy has been reported in nursing children exposed to BZDs, so these drugs should be avoided (27).

## ■ TOBACCO DEPENDENCE

Tobacco is an addicting drug with a definite withdrawal syndrome, familiar to any smoker. Nicotine abstinence is characterized by the *Diagnostic and Statistical Manual of Mental Disorders (Third Edition—Revised)* (28) as being followed by craving for the drug, irritability or anger, anxiety, difficulty in concentration, restlessness, bradycardia, and hyperphagia. Smoking acts to block the effects of withdrawal, which accounts for the reinforcement that cigarettes offer. Nicotine is now available as a gum (Nicorette, 2 mg per square) that blocks most of the withdrawal syndrome, with the notable exception of the craving for cigarettes. Blocking the physical stigmata associated with the withdrawal syndrome facilitates patients working on the psychological reinforcers of smoking. Delivery of the nicotine as a chewing gum allows patients to titrate their level through the vigor of their chewing in a manner analogous to varying the frequency of their cigarettes. Successful treatment depends on instructing the patient on what to realistically expect from the gum. Patients who do well characteristically discontinue the gum within one to two months. Success is greatly facilitated by involvement with a behavioral program as well.

## ■ REFERENCES


1. Greendyke RM, Kanter DR, Schuster DB, et al: Propranolol treatment of assaultive patients with organic brain disease. J Nerv Ment Dis 1986; 174:290-294
2. Yudofsky SC, Silver JM, Schneider SE: Pharmacologic treatment of aggression. Psychiatric Annals 1987; 17:397-402
3. Hakoloa HP, Laulumaa VA: Carbamazepine in treatment of violent schizophrenics. Lancet 1982; 1:1358
4. Luchins DJ: Carbamazepine in violent non-epileptic schizophrenics. Psychopharmacol Bull 1984; 20:569-571
5. Sheard MH, Marini JL, Bridges CJ, et al: The effects of lithium in impulsive aggressive behavior in man. Am J Psychiatry 1976; 33:1409-1413

6. Worrall EP, Moody JP, Naylor GT: Lithium in non-manic depressives: antiaggressive effects and red blood cell lithium values. Br J Psychiatry 1975; 126:464-468
7. Sellers EM, Naranjo CA, Peachey JE: Drugs to decrease alcohol consumption. N Engl J Med 1981; 305:1255-1262
8. Ciraulo DA, Jaffe JH: Tricyclic antidepressants in the treatment of depression associated with alcoholism. J Clin Psychopharmacol 1981; 1:146-150
9. Fawcett J, Clark DC, Aagesen CA, et al: A double-blind, placebo-controlled trial of lithium carbonate therapy for alcoholism. Arch Gen Psychiatry 1987; 44:248-256
10. Rosenbloom AF: Optimizing drug treatment of alcohol withdrawal. Am J Med 1986; 81:901-904
11. Perry JC, Jacobs D: Overview: clinical applications of the amytal interview in psychiatric emergency settings. Am J Psychiatry 1982; 139:552-559
12. Dysken MW, Kooser JA, Haraszti JS: Clinical usefulness of sodium amobarbital interviewing. Arch Gen Psychiatry 1979; 36:789-794
13. Gawin FH: New uses of antidepressants in cocaine abuse. Psychosomatics 1986; 27(supp 11):24-29
14. Halmi KA, Eckert E, LaDu TJ: Anorexia nervosa: treatment efficacy of cyproheptadine and amitriptyline. Arch Gen Psychiatry 1986; 43:177-181
15. Insel TR, Zohar J: Psychopharmacologic approaches to obsessive–compulsive disorder, in Psychopharmacology: The Third Generation of Progress. Edited by Meltzer HY. New York, Raven Press, 1987
16. Stimmel Gl, Escobar JI: Antidepressants in chronic pain: a review of efficacy. Pharmacotherapy 1986; 6:262-267
17. Ward N, Bokan JA, Phillips M, et al: Antidepressants in concomitant chronic back pain and depression: doxepin and desipramine compared. J Clin Psychiatry 1984; 45(sec 2):54-57
18. Davidson J, Raft T: Monoamine oxidase inhibitors in patients with chronic pain. Arch Gen Psychiatry 1985; 42:635-636
19. Charney DS, Woods SW, Goodman WK, et al: Drug treatment of panic disorder: the comparative efficacy of imipramine, alprazolam, and trazodone. J Clin Psychiatry 1986; 47:580-586
20. Gardner DL, Cowdry RW: Positive effects of carbamazepine on behavioral dyscontrol in borderline personality disorder. Am J Psychiatry 1986; 143:519-522
21. Gardner DL, Cowdry RW: Alprazolam-induced dyscontrol in borderline personality disorder. Am J Psychiatry 1985; 142:98-100
22. Soloff PH, George A, Nathan RS, et al: Progress in pharmacotherapy of borderline disorders. Arch Gen Psychiatry 1986; 43:691-697

23. Rieder RO, Rosenthal D, Wender P, et al: The offspring of schizophrenics: fetal and neonatal deaths. Arch Gen Psychiatry 1975; 32:200-211
24. Nurnberg HG, Prudic J: Guidelines for treatment of psychosis during pregnancy. Hosp Comm Psychiatry 1984; 35:67-71
25. Jefferson JW, Greist JH, Ackerman DL, et al: Lithium Encyclopedia for Clinical Practice (second edition). Washington, DC, American Psychiatric Press, 1987
26. Calabrese JR, Golledge AD: Psychotropics during pregnancy and lactation: a review. Psychosomatics 1985; 26:413-426
27. Ananth J: Side effects in the neonate from psychotropic agents excreted through breast feeding. Am J Psychiatry 1978; 135:801-805
28. American Psychiatric Association: Diagnostic and Statistical Manual of Mental Disorders, Third Edition, Revised. Washington, DC, American Psychiatric Association, 1987

# INDEX